Walking with Persephone

A Journey of Midlife Descent and Renewal

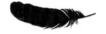

Molly Remer

WOMANCRAFT PUBLISHING

Published by Womancraft Publishing, 2021
www.womancraftpublishing.com

ISBN 978-1-910559-67-3

Walking with Persephone is also available in ebook format: ISBN 978-1-910559-66-6

Cover design, interior design and typesetting: lucentword.com

Cover image © Molly Remer

Womancraft Publishing is committed to sharing powerful new women's voices, through a collaborative publishing process. We are proud to midwife this work, however the story, the experiences and the words are the authors' alone. A percentage of Womancraft Publishing profits are invested back into the environment reforesting the tropics (via TreeSisters) and forward into the community.

The following poems were first published in:
"Persephone Speaks" (Sunlight on Cedar)
"Too Awake" (2020 We'Moon Datebook)
"Persephone Prayersong" (short version in Goddess Devotional)
"Recipe of Wholeness" (Sunlight on Cedar)
"Cliffs of Questioning" (Sunlight on Cedar)
"Prayer for Sacred Pauses" (Goddess Devotional)
"Summer Solstice Blessing" (Whole and Holy)
"Cauldron Prayer" (Goddess Devotional)
"Essential Goodness" (Goddess Devotional)

PRAISE FOR

WALKING WITH PERSEPHONE

What a gloriously contemplative, hopeful, truthful book. It took me deep into my innermost heart and reminded me of the simple grace of being alive. A book to keep nearby when you forget what matters most.

—Jennifer Louden, author of *Why Bother?* and *The Woman's Retreat Book*

Growing up as a high-achiever and a good girl, Molly Remer always did everything she could for everyone else, until it became too much. Her story of "losing her soul" will resonate with many women. She learns that it is necessary to do less for others in order to restore her self.

—Carol P. Christ, author of *Rebirth of the Goddess* and *Goddess and God in the World*

Walking with Persephone opened my heart in such an unexpected way; I felt as though I were having an intimate conversation with a dear friend. Molly's words felt like an echo of my own deepest thoughts and questions and revelations as I have journeyed along the path to middle-age. As I have learned from my many years of leading Red Tent circles, we women need each other's stories in order to understand our own lives. In Walking with Persephone, Molly gifts us all with a powerful and much-needed story of personal transformation and reclamation.

—Amy Wilding, author of *Wild & Wise: Sacred Feminine Meditations for Women's Circles & Personal Awakening*

Packed with Molly Remer's glorious prose and poetry, Walking with Persephone is a heartfelt and glorious read. My copy is furiously marked up with passages to return to. There is much wisdom and healing to be found in this very relatable book.

— Trista Hendren, Creatrix of Girl God Books

I smiled often in recognition while reading Molly Remer's account of her midlife underworld journey, Walking with Persephone. Like her, I find sustenance in my relationship with the natural world, the power of Place, and the Sacred Feminine. I see myself and my community in her story as she meets the challenge of tending to the needs of her inner life while not abandoning responsibilities to family and work. I loved the authenticity of her ruminations; it was like having a heartfelt talk with a good friend. Her words sparked my own creativity as I read, even though midlife is behind me and I grapple with different challenges. All of us will descend and rise time and time again over the course of our lives. I recommend this book as an inspiring map for navigating your own underworld journey, complete with tools and devotional practices to guide you on your way.

— Joanna Powell Colbert, creator of the *Gaian Tarot* and co-creator of *The Herbcrafter's Tarot*

This book is a guide to those who feel torn between the needs of family and community and the needs of their own soul. If you are a lover of solitude who finds herself doing too much, this book is a consolation. While Molly Remer does not offer easy answers, she offers a way forward by staying with the tension in her own life. She roots herself in the natural world, in her fierce belief in everyday magic, in the stories of Persephone, and in daily rituals that will nurture and sustain. And she invites and inspires the reader to do the same. She carefully and honestly explores burnout, overcommitment, and also the tender hope that perhaps the needs of her own soul are not as far off as she may initially think from the life she has so carefully crafted.

— Natalie Bryant Rizzieri, author of *Muddy Mysticism: The Sacred Tethers of Body, Earth and Everyday*

CONTENTS

FALL

To those who feel a nameless longing.
And to Persephone.

If women don't tell our stories and utter our truths in order to chart ways
into sacred feminine experience, who will? It is stories women need. Stories
give us hope, a little guidance, and a lot of bravery.

—Sue Monk Kidd, *Dance of the Dissident Daughter*

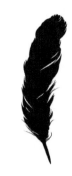

FALL(ING)

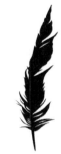

Meeting Persephone

I am unraveling.

Exhausted and depleted. Ragged and worn. I feel as if I am being extinguished, buried under a mountain of too much.

A vision appears, at the edges of sleep and waking, half-dream, half-visualization, images and words, swirling into one.

> *She is shining,*
> *she is shining.*
> *She has come.*
> *She is here.*
> *There are flowers in the ashes*
> *and the hearth is warm again.*

Persephone.

What does a maiden goddess from ancient Greece have to teach middle-aged modern women? What might she teach us about joy and despair, pleasure and pain, depletion and renewal, descent and return?

I am not yet certain, but I do know I have arrived at the gates of the Under-world and stand here shivering, flowers in my hands.

There have been many versions of Persephone's story told over time. Perhaps her story is told and retold in the steps of countless women as they journey through their own lives. Perhaps there are as many walks with Persephone as there are versions of her tale.

The most well-known version of Persephone's story is the ancient Greek myth of a daughter's separation from her mother, her descent into the Underworld, her union with her lover, and her reunion with her mother. In most versions of the tale, Persephone is abducted by the god Hades and transported to the Underworld. Her mother, Demeter, the earth-goddess, searches the land for her daughter and is plunged into grief at the loss. Demeter withholds her nurturing, life-giving powers from the earth, until Persephone returns to her. Meanwhile, Persephone becomes the Queen of the Underworld, guiding lost souls through their passage as they navigate the depths. While in this realm, she eats six pomegranate seeds and then learns that in so doing, she is bound to Hades and to her role as Underworld Queen forever.

Whether the seeds are a metaphorical symbol of her transition into Lover and Queen rather than Maiden, or a literal ingestion that binds her physically to the Underworld, is open to interpretation. The compromise reached, in order to restore the fertility of the earth and to bring it out of an eternal winter, is that Persephone will return to the earth, to Demeter, every spring and spend six months of the year on the earth, bringing about its flourishing and renewal. She will then spend six months in the Underworld, caretaking for those who journey beneath, while the earth rests and prepares for a new season. In this way, Persephone is a goddess of both spring and winter, descent and renewal. She is Maiden, Daughter, Lover, and Queen and, despite the simplicity of her tale, as it is often recounted in brief, it actually means that Persephone is one of the most complex, multi-layered, and multi-faceted goddesses of the Greek era — holding power in multiple realms of existence and in multiple forms of expression. Persephone embodies the full cycle of life. She is whole.

I have been on a goddess-centered path for twenty years. My life's work is wrapped around the creation of small goddess figurines and of the poems and lessons learned from listening to the sacred, to the Goddess in the everyday, as she shows herself to me in myriad small ways — on wings and roses, in clouds and sunbeams, in flashes of insight on the breeze, the rainbow rising above the roof, the swift and languid patterns of the rivers running to the sea, personal and yet impersonal, direct, earthy, and embodied, yet ethereal and wispy, a sensation of knowingness and being held. I have long been centered on the Goddess as a great, grand incarnation of being, the web of life, She Who Holds the Whole, She Who Weaves the All. I perceive her as the fabric of life, the stuff of the universe, that very force which holds the world together. I don't often connect to specific goddesses from other times and places, but rather to the embracing fullness of the Goddess that I feel right here, beneath my feet.

I have hungered for more intense devotional work, for a more direct and personalized connection with a goddess. Despite my familiarity with the many myths and stories of goddess-honoring cultures and practices from around the world, the Goddess for me was just The All, not a distinct and characterized entity, a personalized deity with whom I can experience, dialogue, and directly connect. So when her words and message trailed to me across an urban lake, unexpectedly present, unexpectedly expressed, unexpectedly in communion with something specific, I wondered: *Why Persephone, why now?*

To experience Persephone directly, embodied, incarnate, present, characterized, personalized, personified, was a surprise. It was something that I thought, perhaps, was not possible for me, was not meant to be a part of my own spiritual experience.

I first read the story of Persephone when I was in my early twenties, beginning my first deep dive into the literature of feminist spirituality. I read the feminist reinterpretation of the tale by Charlene Spretnak when I trained as a *Cakes for the Queen of Heaven* facilitator at age twenty-eight. In this version, Persephone consciously and deliberately separates from her mother, seeking her independence and then willingly accepts Hades into her arms and bed as a devoted lover. In still other versions, reputed to be earlier translations, Hades is not involved at all, but rather Persephone hears the cries of the dead reverberating from the Underworld and goes to their aid.

Persephone is too girlish, too out of control of her own fate, too maiden-like for me to identify with her at first. She is too flowery and, dare I say, maybe even seems "weak" and powerless. In fact, the year that the large goddess festival held each year in the neighboring state of Kansas chooses Persephone as the goddess to honor, I skip it, saying that I don't really connect. I return instead when they work with The Morrigan, She of the crows and wild ferocity.

It isn't until much later, long after my walk with Persephone begins and after the first draft of this manuscript is already complete, that I read a quote from Sue Monk Kidd in her book *Traveling with Pomegranates* (co-authored with daughter Ann Kidd Taylor):

To borrow a phrase from Dylan Thomas, Persephone is the "green fuse" in the soul, the regenerative energy. She's the bright, invisible sap within that must rise after fifty.

Yes. This is the Persephone I have come to know. The persistent, the insistent, the rising from within, the fiery core of resolve that cannot be quenched.

Laura Sims, writing in her essay "A New Telling of the Myth" in the Demeter and Persephone anthology *The Long Journey Home,* describes the power of living into a story and myth in the present:

> *The story is an initiation, holding within it obvious and secret instructions about becoming fully alive in one's body, on the earth, and in the universe. [...] Within the images, like seeds that have preserved their origins within the husk, inspiration can be summoned that stimulates authentic awakening and growth toward a greater sense of interdependence and bliss in the world.*

My purpose, when I started writing what was to become this book, was to explore what it means to intentionally rebuild my soul as a midlife woman without leaving my commitments, my family, or my work, somehow discovering how to stoke my own fire, how to feed my own flame, and how to tend to my own heart with primacy and care, while at the same time doing the other things that *really matter.* As I began this conscious and intentional process of deconstructing and re-constructing my life, the goddess Persephone entered my world and I began a process of walking with her on an intensive path of discovering, uncovering, and remembering who I am and how I wish to live my life.

It seems that it is the path of my story, the elements of my journey, that brought her rising in my consciousness to meet me. There are mythic connections woven throughout time and space, themes that connect modern experiences to ancient places, timeworn stories that have become faded and threadbare, missing pieces to reconstruct, but still carrying a timeless wisdom for the journey of living.

I have a sense that whilst the details of my walk with Persephone were personal, the themes and many of the elements are universal to women traveling the path of midlife. I offer it to you as a companion to the journey, a travel guide for the Underworld process of rebuilding your soul. I hope it is of comfort as you take your own steps into the known and unknown, becoming more alert to the signs, symbols, and messages in your everyday life in an everyday world and discovering the magic and mysticism that are right there in your own backyard.

Circle

The sacred space beneath your feet
requires no self-flagellation,
no stain of desperation
on your skin.
The wind across your brow
sees no need for shame.
Your own holy worth
is beyond question.
Despair is not the price you pay
to live this life,
to hear this truth,
to feel this
love.

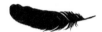

I gather with a circle of powerful women in a log house on a hill, overlooking a deep meadow. The sky is heavy with rain, tolling sorrowfully and heavily across the land. The landscape of being within our circle is also heavy and tearful. Pain and struggle are waiting below the surface of each woman in the circle, waiting, waiting, waiting for a safe space in which to be expressed.

It has been three months since we last circled together and it is easy to see how we have missed this outlet for expression and connection. After we sing a promise of sanctuary to one another, the tears begin, the secrets of our lives brought forward, and we learn that our shames and our sufferings are not solitary experiences after all. After each woman's turn with the rattle, we note that the sky reflects our mood, hanging gray and somber, heavy and full of emotion, wet with tears, overflowing our banks, flooding through us.

When it is my turn with the rattle, I break into tears as I attempt to articulate the crossroads of life at which I find myself. In a recent poem, I wrote that my work is:

To be both not enough and too much simultaneously and to sit in the middle
of both and just be okay. Because that is all that I have.

That is all that I have, I almost shout into the silent witnessing of the circle. And that is true.

I am nearly forty. I have been in the same relationship for twenty-four years. I am feeling an insistent call that it is *time for something to change.* I feel brittle. Worn. Taut. Sharp-edged. Thin. Flickering. Parched and hungry. At the verge of tears often. I feel as if I only like myself when I'm alone and I am *so rarely alone.* I have a craving for solitude that sometimes makes me feel as if I will die from the longing. I feel a knowing within myself that I can either consciously choose to deconstruct and rebuild my own life or that something will happen that will make the choice for me.

I feel as if I have been piling things into my arms for the last twenty years, holding it all, managing it all, doing it all, being it all and suddenly I am looking at the pile, realizing how much of it doesn't belong to me, and hungering to let it drop, to lay it all down, to walk away. I have learned that when people see you carrying a lot and not dropping anything, they often think, *I guess she can hold this for me.* When they see you saying yes, they decide to also ask you for things. When they see you doing something, they think, *She can do something for me too.* And, eventually, the load becomes unbearable and you are driven into the ground by a weight that you have opened your arms to accept.

> *I want to shed obligation and to deprogram my "could" reflex.*
> *I want to soak in my own knowing and stoke my own well-being.*
> *I want to learn how to hold my center in the*
> *middle of everything and still be okay.*
> *I want to tend to my friendships with love and*
> *compassion and to tend to my marriage, but mainly*
> *I want to tend to my own weary heart.*
> *I am ready to look at what I've been carrying and let go*
> *of what isn't mine. I am ready to restructure, rebirth,*
> *renew, rediscover, re-evaluate, reconsider, refill, refuel, and*
> *rebuild. I am ready to write myself back into being.*
> *I am starting from now.*

I am starting from here.
I am starting.
I will rebuild my wholeness, my connections,
my devotion, my heart.
I want to taste my life and love the flavor.
I want to drink deeply of the magic of being.

I tell the women in the Red Tent that I am going to do an experiment. I tell them I don't feel like sharing it yet, but that I know what it is.

The Experiment

This morning, I step out of the back door and three deer leap away through the woods, long white tails flashing in the gray morning. One picks her way more slowly across the stones, the same stones on which I stand each morning. The cry of a hawk rings in the air. A woodpecker settles into its morning work. As I step onto the stones myself, a lone crow arcs overhead, traveling to join its family, who I can hear calling from our compost pile in the woods, near the other side of the house. These are the rhythms I am born from. These are the moments of being that sustain me. This is what I want more of in my days.

The experiment, this experiment of rebuilding the richness of my life, of letting this magic I know of weave through me and fuel my soul, will take this form:

I will visit the woods every day and write down what I learn.
I will go for a walk every day, in as many
new, small backyard journeys as I can.
I will watch for messages.
I will be alert for signs.
I will be open to as much magic as I can be.
I will redefine and minimize my time on social media.

I will restructure and renegotiate my work schedule and work life.
I will trust myself.
I will allow myself to feel.
I will ask myself what I want, really want, and I will do that.
I will let projects, things, and people go.
I will read the books I want to read and I will sink into
my own life and rebuild the practices that sustain me.
I will remember that I am a conduit for the holy.
I will walk in the hand of the Goddess and
let her love me back into myself.
I will walk on the land, kneel on the stones, listen to the
flowers, learn from the trees, and sing with the river.
I will say no as much as possible, so that I
can have room to laugh again.
I will stand up for my own needs and rights.
I will walk away.
I will walk toward.
I will claim my own powers.
I will allow my own magic to well up and sing through my veins.
I will claim myself.
I will go to bed when I want to.
I will pee when I need to.
I will lie on the floor and let the tightness in my
back and shoulders melt into the earth.
I will know myself as whole and worthy and capable,
but capable will no longer define me as
my primary reason for being.
I will listen. Truly listen.
To my soul.
I will wander and wonder and uncover what I know
as I explore the terrain both within and without,
with tender, fierce commitment and depth.
I will coax my own truth out of hiding.
I will allow myself the opportunity to experience daily delight.
I will give myself time. Great, wide swaths of beautiful time.
I will defragment my brain and re-weave my spirit.

Mark and I go for a walk before dinner. We set off around the field, a cleared and sloping hillside, blanketed with the golden rays of bluestem grasses. One of my favorite experiences in recent months has been to watch the way the sunset filters through the glistening puffs of seed fluff on these grasses and to delight in their color as they glow in the twilight. Tonight, however, the sky remains heavy and gray, but three deer at the crest of the hill turn and run into the woods, white flags of their tails waving farewell. Then, a lone crow traces a path through the sky, quietly swooping, though we hear the raucous cries of its family echoing up from the river bottom. I am struck by how my day has been bookended by my two walking experiences, three deer and a crow.

I am here.

I am listening.

Our breathing is heavy with exertion and there is not much need for conversation. After our circuit up the hill and around the field, we admire the imposing cliff face that nestles somewhat unobtrusively amongst the trees. It is steep and massive, a beautiful rock formation that really only catches your eye when you stand in its shadow and look up, lurking mysteriously and quietly there above you, needing no acknowledgment, simply existing, and yet with an undeniable, palpable sensation of solid presence. There is a mossy boulder beneath it in the field, carpeted with soft green. A thick grapevine arches over it as if to make a gateway into the Otherworld. As I stand my small goddess figures in this tiny world of moss and vine, Mark points out that the boulder was once a part of the cliff we have been admiring, toppling from its perch and coming to rest many feet below, perhaps thousands of years before we stand here, in the dusk, noticing the moss and feeling our feet on the earth.

We are silent for a moment, appreciating this reality, this smallness and this bigness all rolled together in one mossy pinpoint of life.

I look at the thick cord of grapevine forming an arch over the boulder blanketed with moss and feel the sensation, *this is it.* In a good way. A rich, deep, holy and sacred way. I need the experience of discovery, of awe, and wonder, *every day.*

How might I expand my sensation of enchanted, magical living out from the slender margins and into the fullness of my hours and how I live? I can taste it, glimpse it, yes, but can I wholeheartedly embody and embrace it as primary? Can I consciously, intentionally, mindfully, weave my life out of sticks and stones and moss and words?

The Crows

My word of the year is *listen.* I order it stamped on metal disk and fasten the disk to one of our goddess figurines along with a crow charm.

I am going to listen to the crows.

Crows are plentiful in our area, but they have a particular way of catching my eye and my attention. I often wake to the sound of crows outside my bedroom window. One even woke me on a winter's morning by dropping a composted baked potato skin, frozen solid, onto the roof of our house, where it rolled end over end to land with a thud on the back deck in a slightly accusatory fashion *(better snacks are in order, lady!).*

I watch them perching observantly in the trees above the compost pile. I spot them in the air, in fields, and on fence posts and trees while driving. While I don't always know exactly what the crows are saying, I know to pay attention to them and to listen. I have often experienced them as an answer to a question, a message from the Goddess, and even just as a reminder of the simple magic in the air.

The sound or sight of a crow is always a sign for me to stop and pay attention — it becomes a self-reinforcing encounter with everyday magic. The crow is a trigger for me — listen, watch, look here, reflect, think, feel, experience, *be here right now.* And in so stopping, I often see or experience something magical, surprising, or significant. Whether or not magic is there already (out of my awareness) or it is merely the simple association with the crow as a sign to pay attention which causes me to look more closely and to develop associations, make connections, or notice symbols and make significance out of the mundane world, the end result is the same — I pause, notice, encounter, and experience, and the encounter itself *becomes magic* in that act of noticing and experiencing.

Crows have been associated with dark goddesses for millennia, particularly with The Morrigan, the ferocious Celtic Goddess-Queen of the battlefield. They are also associated with magic, prophecy, mysticism, death, and the Underworld. For me, they are a powerful symbol of everyday magic, a touchstone with spirit on the wing. Increasingly, though not reflected in ancient myths, over the course of this year, these clever black birds become a sign of Persephone to me: her answer to my questions, a breath of mystery over my shoulder, a nod, a nudge, an affirmation, a direct reply, a message above my head. Each crow—and especially three crows in a row—that I encounter feels like a connection with the Goddess, a connection to Persephone, the way in which she is speaking to me as my story labors into life.

Is it just a crow or is it Goddess on the wing, magic in the air, the weaving of life itself laid black against the sky? These crows guide the way into the next part of my own story, the next moment of meaning, and shape how I understand myself, my spirituality, and the everyday enchantment of the world itself. There are few things that set me back down into my bones again as firmly and insistently as a crow—present and witnessing, alert and alive, hopeful and inspired, aware and open.

In *Burning Woman*, Lucy H. Pearce writes:

For some she came in a dream. For others in words as clear as a bell: it is time, I am here. She may come in a whisper so loud she can deafen you or a shout so quiet you strain to hear. She may appear in the waves or the face of the moon, in a red goddess or a crow.

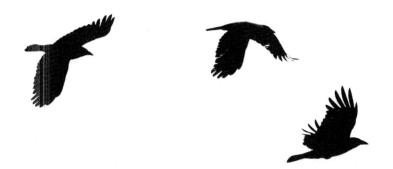

Crows are dark goddess symbols of myth, legend, prophecy, meaning, and mysticism. They are commonplace and ordinary and yet show up at exactly the right moment and in unexpected ways in flashes of acknowledgment. They have become part of the language of the divine to me, the way the Goddess speaks in the world. I like reclaiming dangerous symbols and reverting them back into symbols of power and magic, instead of fear or bad omens. The Goddess herself was nearly lost beneath negative imagery, associations, and accusations and crows too, gathered in murders as they do, have suffered from loss of reputation too—the subverting of their magic into something uneasy and mistrusted. So, I call my spirit back on the wings of crows. I call magic back on the wings of crows. I invite everyday magic and mysticism to enliven my days and it arrives on the wings of crows. I invite the Goddess to speak to and through me and she speaks with crows.

I came to associate crows, hawks, and vultures—all three—with Persephone on this journey, even though, mythically speaking, only vultures have any association—and that is with Hades. Very often a crow, and often three crows, would appear in answer to my questions, bookend my insights, or respond to my prayers or pleas. When I speak to Persephone and then look up to see a crow, I've come to understand that I've been heard.

A life lesson is often dished up to us directly, just waiting to be seen. If you see your life through the lens of story, you can watch, perceive, and notice when the next part is being written—crows *are* that for me, the indicator of presence, of paying attention, of writing it all home and into being, soul, and form.

This is My Real Life

When I feel a lull in my work today, I listen to my own impulse to step outside, instead of pushing through or opening apps on my phone. I follow the path to the stones in the woods and step out onto them. It is colder than I expected. The slender maple trees are gray and the sky continues to hang in a gray bowl, overturned on top of a leafless forest.

As I stand there waiting, a single crow flies across the treeline to my right. It is silent, though I can hear other crows calling from a distance. It crests the trees and begins to circle and wheel on widespread black wings in the open sky above the valley. It coasts, barely ever moving its wings, much like a vulture coasts, in widening and then narrowing circles on invisible currents of air. I feel like a witness to a dance. I wonder at the perspective offered by soaring on open wings. I wonder what I can learn from this graceful, coasting presence soaring above me. Long moments pass and then the crow drops out of my line of sight into the forest.

For a brief moment, the sky, the trees, and the air all feel completely still. I feel still too. My breath and mind slow, bearing witness to this quiet crow-dance.

Then, I feel lucky—how fortunate that I stepped out at exactly this moment, otherwise I would have missed the dance completely. What if I hadn't followed my impulse, hadn't seen this? I wonder how many other moments of magic I miss, indoors each day. Perhaps this exact moment, this exact experience, this exact dance, was at some level meant for me to see.

When I step back onto the back deck, I hear the distant chorus of wild geese in the air and more crows begin to call. A blue jay squawks and soars over my right shoulder to land in a nearby tree. I squint into the gray, but still bright sky and see the geese. There are five V-formations of them, high above me, a steady stream of sound issuing from them as they journey by.

When I return indoors, I feel altered somehow. I have long said that when I need to feel magic in my life, I go outside and look for a bird. This year, that element of magic seems heightened more than ever. I feel like I have discerned my task at last:

> *to listen*
> *and live from*
> *the story*
> *of my life*
> *writing itself*
> *right now.*

I teach a writing class at our homeschool co-op and I encourage the teenagers in my class to experiment with writing non-fiction stories about their own lives as well as fiction.

You have to believe you have a story worth telling, I say to them.

And, despite my own questioning and my own state of exploration, I do believe I have a story worth telling and that sustains me. I live in a storied reality, and these stories shape me and my understanding of myself, the world, and my place in it. I look for the stories of my life each day.

What if I just watch the magic unfold around me every day and write about that, I wonder. No going backwards into time and trying *to figure it out,* or convince anyone of anything. What if I view my life as a storied reality to learn from *as it is being written* — to write myself into form and look for the writing of life as it is lived? I will tell what is actually happening, learn from it, explain and process and connect the ideas and experiences from it, as they unfold this very year.

Writing this book will be the first time I've worked on something with a sustained, day-by-day effort that I haven't then shared right away in some form or another. I started blogging in 2006 and everything I write, minus personal journal entries, has usually been written for relatively immediate "consumption" or distribution. This time, I'm holding something close to my heart and seeing where it takes me, writing myself into form, writing my life into story, writing the shape of my soul into being.

I continue to write for several hours. I become aware that my shoulders are tight, my head is beginning to ache, and my heart feels like it is beating too fast. Instead of pushing through these physical cues, I recognize them as signs that I need to take a break.

I move a *lot* of energy through me on Mondays, the day in which I am left completely alone to work. A lot of creative energy bubbles up from me and I produce a lot of work that then sustains and fuels me through the rest of the week. On the heels of such an energetically intense Red Tent circle, it almost feels like more than I can handle, or more than I can continue to process and integrate right now.

I head back outside and walk to the field in front of the house. There, I kneel on golden bluestem grasses, placing both my hands onto the earth. Though it is cold out, the ground feels warm beneath my hands. I feel an urge to lie down, stretched flat upon the ground, the way I used to do as a girl, at those times when I experienced sudden moments of expanded consciousness, feeling exquisitely aware of the whole world spinning beneath me.

I don't lie down, for some reason, though. I wonder what would have happened during the rest of the day if I would have done so. Instead, I hear the call of a lone crow and look up to see it flying in the trees nearby. I feel a sensation of delight and amazement again that bubbles up in my chest: *this is it. This is my real life!* And then, the sound of wild geese again, this time too high in the clouds for my eyes to reach them.

When I come back inside, I put peppermint oil on my neck and temples and lie stretched out flat on the floor for a few minutes, rather than immediately continuing my work. As I lie there, deep guttural moans emerge from me, the primal type of sounds of a woman giving birth. Instead of silencing myself, I let them out and feel oddly satisfied.

Perhaps these acts do not sound radical, but I believe they are. I do not often give myself permission to simply lie on the floor and this urge, so often denied, starts to become the heart of my most dominant fantasies. Part of the rebuilding of my life needs to include ample opportunities to lie on the floor.

A Goddess Path

I began walking a goddess path in an academic sense about twenty years ago—academic meaning reading, thinking, evaluating, and making an intentional and conscious socio-political statement of values about the role and power and value of women's bodies, stories, and lives. Goddess spirituality was academic and mental for me at first, something I thought about and it *made sense* for me. Goddess as a concept made sense, Goddess as a statement made sense, Goddess as a revolution made sense, and Goddess as a radical affirmation of the feminist values I held—the power of something wildly different than the dominant, patriarchal, monotheistic conception of divinity.

Sixteen years ago, I began making goddess art. Pregnant with my first baby, my thealogy* moved from the academic and into the practical, becoming very embodied, earthy, centered in the body and the physical, lived realities of being in form. Goddess, for me, became connected to the embodied experiences of pregnancy, birthing, nursing, and parenting. For a long time, I worked only with the Goddess in this way—as a broad, numinous, ineffable presence, the Great She, She who holds the universe together, the great, grand, glorious whole, the weaving of the world itself.

Most of my work since has been born from this understanding. With time,

---

* Thealogy is the study of the Goddess, as well as the exploration of the meaning of Goddess symbols historically and currently. It includes exploration of the embodied, relational experience of Goddess and is a visioning of Divinity through a feminist lens. Thealogy helps us to answer the question posed by thealogian Dr. Shirley Ann Ranck of, "what would it have been like to grow up in a world with the divine imagined as female…" through studying Goddess legacies from ancient cultures as well as forming a new worldview based on feminist principles *and* on direct, embodied, personal experiences with the sacred feminine.

I came to see that there are also distinct, individual goddesses within the great, grand weaving: sovereign in their own rights, each one a thread in the tapestry of the whole. I feel like it is possible to sense these goddesses and to reach through the web to touch the thread that is the specific goddess you are working with—the thread of distinct and sovereign presence that is Brigid, is Durga, is Kuan Yin, is Persephone, is Hecate.

When I discovered goddess spirituality, I felt almost driven to try to prove the existence of the Goddess in the world, to convince others of the value of this path, to share my new understandings and delighted "enlightenment" with others.

I have been described by friends as a "born educator" and even when I was a homeschooled child, playing "public school" with my friends, I was always the teacher. At the beach this past winter, walking with Mark, I told him that I no longer feel as if I have anything to teach. I just want to tell people about the shell I found today. This feels true at a deep level. I no longer feel a hunger or compulsion to try to convince anyone of anything, to try to change anyone's mind, to try to make my case, or prove my point. Now, I realize, I was still in a process of proving something to myself, of doggedly, devotedly discovering myself as a spiritual being and forming a relationship with the spiritual forces and presences around me.

I don't need to prove Her to anyone anymore. She has woven herself into being right in front of me in countless, myriad, magical, enchanting ways and I no longer need to explain, justify, rationalize, or prove her existence in my life.

I know that some readers may be looking for a series of steps to invite the Goddess in, to witness her magic, to feel her hands in their lives. What does it *mean* to work with a specific goddess, to walk with a specific goddess, and how do you find this relationship if you crave it, but don't have it?

One way to connect is to study—to read, to contemplate, to learn about goddess spirituality, about specific goddesses, to meditate on the goddesses, to do divination, to ask for dreams, to freewrite in your journal, to consciously open yourself up to the presence of a goddess and to be alert for signs, signals, symbols and how they connect to what you are studying and learning.

Another way to connect is through dedicated devotional practice. For more than a decade before I began working directly with Persephone, I maintained a daily practice of devotion to the great, grand incarnation of the Goddess, as she who weaves the whole, she who holds the whole. I dedicated specific practices to her—song, prayer, breath, openness, alertness, writing. A prayer practice, a meditation practice, a flame-keeping practice, an altar tending practice... each of these can connect you and root you in a living experience and expression of goddess spirituality. Practices of sound, song, adornment, movement, bathing, and ritual can also help you to bring an experience of the Goddess into your life. If you would like more structured guidance, I have shared more at the end of the book.

I caution you against looking at goddess spirituality as a cookbook or a buffet line, where you pick a goddess that looks appealing and then *boom* now she's *your* goddess and you work with her. I caution against picking and choosing among goddesses or using them for different reasons as if they are treats to be sampled or ingredients for a recipe—need compassion, just stir in one scoop of Kuan Yin—rather than embarking on a process of unfolding, of dedication, and discovery. However, perhaps it really can be so simple and if your relationship with and to the goddess in your life feels simple and easy that doesn't mean that you're doing it wrong, because this is not a path with rules or absolutes.

When considering a specific goddess to work with, consider too that her story has likely been stripped of most of its power and essence and pared back, as a means of reinforcing a social structure or moral lesson of the day, or it has been boiled down from a more complex presence into only a single aspect. It is worth bearing in mind that whilst Greek goddess names are often familiar to us in popular culture and modern experience, Greek tales are often extremely misogynistic and patriarchal in approach. So whilst the names themselves are accessible, I would like to also point out that I view these as newer representations of much older powers, more ancient goddess identities with more to offer than the Wikipedia version of the goddess.

I do know that for me, it has not rested on intellectualizing or even ritualizing, but rather in *showing up,* showing up in fear, doubt, confusion, pain, joy, anger, suffering, triumph and in devotion, in listening to and seeing what is right before my eyes. For me, it is a multi-layered, complex, nuanced, winding and indeed, more *binding* process.

Until this walk with Persephone emerged into my life, in which her story, lessons, and symbols came alive in my world as a lived and living reality, much of my work with Goddess was in a metaphoric and symbolic sense, rather than in the grit and dirt of living... Sometimes the way you know that what you are doing or experiencing is *real* is that the goddess chooses you and your experience of her is different than what you might have cognitively planned for, hoped for, or imagined.

I woke with her in my mind
under my skin
below my thoughts,
and him, too, in the shadows.
and there was the shining
again and again
the sensation that she is coming,
she is coming
she is coming,
she is here
and in the dark corners,
the dark caves,
the dark caverns,
there is light,
there is a blazing,
there is a brilliance
from her that illuminates
and in the hearth, grown cold
and full of ashes,
bright flowers bloom and flare
and blaze and twine
from ashes across cracked stones
illuminated by her glow,
by her radiance,
a flame among shadows,
she walks
and darkness crumbles away.
She is fed from within,
shining from inside,
illuminated with love and she glows
how she glows,
with passion and power and creation.

There is honey on her tongue,
flowers in her hair,
love in her eyes,
music in her voice.
She is shining,
she is shining.
She has come,
she is here.
There are flowers in the ashes
and the hearth is warm again.

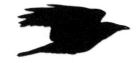

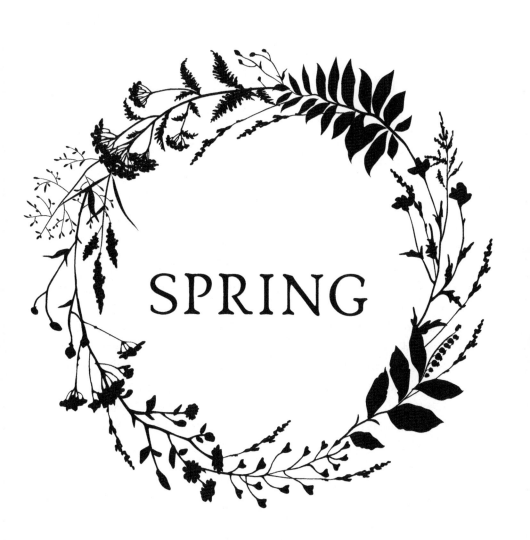

SPRING

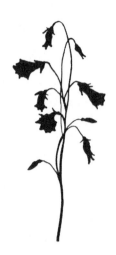

MARCH

The Work Begins Today

The morning dawns gray and cold again. As I step out onto the rocks, I feel the welcome sensation of magic lingering here. It is unfailing. I felt it the first time I stepped here and I have felt it every day since.

I breathe deep as I step off into the slender young maple trees, their trunks as gray as the sky and I think, *I need more of this.* I find a hollow stump, ringed with bright moss and nestle a goddess in the leaves filling the hollow. I sit on a damp stone and this time I think, *how can I feel this more often?* Thunder rumbles over my left shoulder and crows call to the right and the answer comes, so simple and obvious that it is clear it *isn't* from me: *to feel this more often, just **do** this more often.*

This is what I will do. This is what I need.

I look out at the horizon and two crows swoop into my line of vision on the left, heading for the gray open sky over the field. A pause and a quiet falls over the forest and then a third crow, swoops in from the right side calling out loudly as it heads off to join the others. As I sit, looking after them, I feel a sensation of warmth and delight filling me, though the wind is chilly, the branches bare, and the sky gray. This is one of my answers, I feel it in my body.

The work begins today.

My Womanrunes card* for the day is the Circle, the rune of oneself. I feel starved for myself lately, craving my own companionship, thirsting for the opportunity to think and to feel and to listen and learn from my very own self. I continue to ponder how I might hold my center in the midst of the swirl, how to connect with the Goddess when people are clamoring all around me, how to replenish my spirit when I am drained by human contact and continuous companionship.

At homeschool co-op, after teaching two classes, I head for the park across the street: its lake is calling to me. I have determined I will make friends with this lake this year. Two wild geese are on the shore, placidly rooting around in the heavily rain-saturated soil. A dead goose floats amongst the litter at the lake's edge. I see robins and hear red-winged blackbirds. The wind is so wild that there are waves in the lake, lapping at the shore, which is bordered by numerous knobby bumps of roots.

I find a bowl of roots in which to nestle a goddess figure and I lean back on the solid trunk of what I think is a cedar tree. There is loud, incongruous music playing from a nearby construction site, but there is wildness here too, I feel it. I feel like the lake is responding to me and sending me a gift. The wind is whipping, swirling my hair up and around my face and chilling my bare arms, my feet sink into the squelchy ground. Raindrops splatter my cheeks and nose and the small urban waves lap insistently at the shoreline, into those fascinating cragged and twisted root formations. I, too, feel wild, secret, unbound, alone in my witnessing of these irreplaceable moments of life unfolding constantly whether or not I can be bothered to pause to notice them.

I offer myself up to this initiatory process:

May I be cleansed, renewed, and rebirthed.

---

* Womanrunes are a female-identified oracle system and symbolic language of divine guidance originally created in the 1980s by Shekhinah Mountainwater that I expanded and developed in 2014. For more see my book *Womanrunes: Interpretation Guide.*

May I gain wider perspective and a depth of vision.
May I clear out stagnant patterns and processes.
May I be open, receptive, and flowing.

I hear an answer in the breeze, or in my mind:

You don't know what the lessons will look like
Or how long they will last,
But you will know them when you see them.

I take my hands from my coat pockets and hold them open. I feel a distinct sensation of cool air filling my palms like two balls of energy and my breath puffs out in a cloud carried away into the sunlight.

I am ready.

The First Task

My Womanrune of the day today is the Hearth, rune of nurturance and domesticity, but also the "codependency trap." I find myself reflecting on my relationship with my family and my work and how often family obligations and commitments are used in subtly shaming ways by internet memes in either an effort to encourage women to "stay small" and not have too high expectations for themselves or almost as an excuse for our own inabilities to achieve our own dreams, as a reason to hold ourselves back.

I think of messages such as: *Who will be at your hospital bedside? Not the people who read your books or attended your classes, but your family, who you didn't have enough time for, while you were pursuing your teaching/writing/whatever.* I think of well-meaning, but poorly timed, *You'll miss this,* comments to mothers of melting-down toddlers.

I have been parenting for fifteen years and I *still want both.* I want meaningful work, I want to make a broader difference in the world, *and* I want deep, fulfilling, harmonious connections with my own family. I don't think we should be expected to choose between them or to consider these two aspects of life to be mutually exclusive purposes, intentions, values, and commitments. At the same time, here I sit, feeling stretched, worn, and thin from "doing it all." Something *does* need to change in the work-life balance and structure I've created for myself. I want to have more fun. I want to laugh more often. I want to snuggle longer. I want to play more. I want to rest more.

> *The first task*
> *in rebuilding*
> *your soul*
> *is to allow*
> *a wide margin*
> *for magic.*

Initiation with Air

I wake each morning with a prayer on my lips and sometimes a song in my head. It is my daily practices that fuel and sustain me, they rebuild my soul anew each morning, giving me inspiration and sustenance to carry me through the day.

As I write, I remember a moment from five years ago. I was musing in the woods on how to know that I'm really speaking to the Goddess, how to know that this is *real,* that I'm not making it up or talking to an imaginary friend. I was recording my thoughts, as I often do, on my phone's voice memos feature, in a sense channeling the words of the Goddess through me. *Is it her, or is it "only me,"* I wonder at times. I am asking, *Who do I speak to out here?* and I am told that I speak to Gaia: *Goddess of the Woods. Earth Mother. Star Mother. Divine Mother.*

> I *live here. And you are an opening for my words. You touch deep magic here. Ancient, ancient, ancient, vibrant reality. The web waited for you. It sings for you and through you and with you. I*

called your name. I guided you to this place. And I invited you to hear my voice. Dialog is possible, change is possible, healing is possible. You need me and I need you.

At then at this very moment, as I speak and listen, a snake enters my line of sight moving through the leaves. It raises its head and looks at me and we are eye-to-eye for a timeless, holy, powerful, potent moment of communion and message.

I have the exact moment on my audio recording. My voice suddenly stops and there is silence and a long pause and then I just say, *Wow!* I could hardly believe that this moment happened, that this is my real life. That I asked and was answered in such an undeniably clear way. After this experience, I rarely doubt Her again.

This morning, I stand on the rocks listening to the crows, wondering if they are always there, or if we just keep the same schedule. I can't see them, I just hear their voices. I feel heavy and burdened by the to-dos of the day. Our employees will arrive in a few minutes, but I am starting to recognize in myself that I really, really need fewer people in my house on fewer days. Just as I hear and honor this for myself, a crow slides into view to my right, silent black wings carrying it quickly out of sight into the valley where another crow that I hadn't realized was there, dives out of an oak tree to join it. A beat of a pause and then the third crow too, silent black wingbeats carrying it to the others, all sinking out of my line of vision into the valley below.

Three crows in morning.

The wind whips around, striking my face with cold sharpness. The trees are gray and stark. I miss the green. I feel cut through by the wind. I feel hollowed out. I feel dry and parched, thirsty for myself. I need to rededicate myself, I think. I check into the current of my life, the river of feeling that runs below the surface of it — *is there any joy still there?* I am pleased to find that there is still joy there, a wellspring of it, just below the parched and cracked surface, but I also sense that something is starting to block my access to it. I feel separated, like a dam is being built: the wellspring is there, but I may not be able to reach it for much longer. Abruptly, the wind stills and silence falls briefly throughout the whole woods. I feel a sensation of renewal, of rebirth, of baptism by Air.

As I turn to go back inside, I realize I hear no more sound from the crows. They *aren't* always there in the same place all day doing the same thing, but our rhythms do intersect at predictable times. This comforts me.

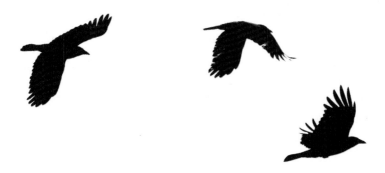

We take our evening walk along our gravel road, stopping to look at mushrooms, stumps, and stones that appear to be miniature landscapes, cliffs to be scaled and worlds to be explored. We make our way home across the neighboring field, golden with bluestem grasses and dotted with cow pies and brambles.

Halfway up the hill, we stop to watch a vulture playing in the updraft. Again, the ragged wings look like a kite to me. At first we think it is a bald eagle, which admittedly would be cooler, but then we see the telltale red head of the turkey vulture. This lone wind-dancer is soon joined by a second and they wheel lazily in a wide circle, we never see either one of them flap their wings, they are just coasting on the currents of air. We watch them for several long moments. The sky is bright and blue again, the full sun still shining in the West with only small dots of white clouds. *I know this isn't the same as seeing an eagle, but I might have something to learn from these too,* I tell Mark. We continue ascending the hill and at the top, before we climb back over the fence, I find a gift lying in the grass. The long, slender, gray-brown wing feather of a vulture. This is the first vulture feather I've ever found or touched. I feel a little twinge of creepiness from the find, but I also think of my moments in the woods this morning with the wind and I think about the crows and the wild geese and I know:

This is part of my (re) initiation with Air.

In fact, what I have just told Mark on this very walk? That I feel charred and on the verge of being extinguished, that I need to rebuild my soul with the practices that sustain me. The vulture is a symbol of cleansing and renewal. In fact, as we gazed up into the impossibly tall, still, leafless sycamore trees over the flooded road, I also said: *I really love this world.* I do, and I must bear witness to these moments of unfolding or the charred sensation will creep further into me and I will lose what I most value.

I set the feather in the hollowed out top of a fence post as I climb over the fence and right inside the post, I find a loose twig, covered with the soft buds of new growth.

At the end of the driveway, watching the sun set behind the neighbor's oak trees, we hear a soft hooting call. I think it is an owl at first, but then I say it is probably actually a mourning dove. Shortly after I speak, a mourning dove flies out of the tree near me, followed a few seconds later by its mate. *I need this,* I tell Mark, *I need to be here watching the world. This is what I live for.* He kisses me quietly and we watch the last sliver of sun drop beneath the trees.

The Second Task

This morning there is a layer of frost on the porch and a chill in the air. My breath makes a cloud by my face as I follow the path of moss and stone into the woods. The black cat twines around my ankles as I gaze out to the horizon line. I hear at least five distinct woodpeckers this morning and see two of different species. Two crows swoop by on the right as I have expected them to do. I wait for the third, but I only hear it and don't see another.

The sky is blue and clear today, no more gray, and I can see sun — rich, glorious, glittering, beautiful, life-giving sun! It filters through the cedar branches in a way that never fails to captivate me. The air is quiet today, the wind has settled and stilled. I feel cleared out and clean and I make a promise, a prayer, a vow: *I will learn from Air.*

When I get back to the porch, I turn to greet the rising sun and offer my daily prayers. I hear a bird and I think: *There! It is that third crow! Such magic!*

But, it is actually one of the mourning doves, settling onto an oak branch in front of me and calling to her mate, who answers her.

> *The second task*
> *is to learn*
> *from Air [and the elements].*

Three Snail Shells (On the Right Path)

In the late afternoon, before dinner, we decide to go on quick ramble on the bluff by Lost Creek. This water- and time-worn sculpture of stone is awe-inspiring and powerful to behold. It looks like it should be a landmark, a state park, a place to visit and climb and explore, but due to its location and the tree line, it is actually nearly invisible until you're standing just below it. It isn't even possible to photograph it very clearly. It has shelves of overhanging rock, many pockets, cavities, chambers, and tiny caverns that make it appear to be a cliff-dwelling city for gnomes. We see two vultures, high above us. I feel my affinity for their wisdom and respect for their contribution to the planet growing stronger each day, though I'm still not positive what I'm supposed to be learning from them.

As we skitter back down the steep hillside, feet sliding in the dark, leaf-strewn soil, holding onto small dogwood and redbud trees for support, we find three snail shells. I laugh that our homing instinct to find shells is so powerful that we can even find them in a forest. Spiral shells, usually cherished beach finds, will always be a sign that we're on the right path, going the right direction.

> *Tread carefully.*
> *Tread lightly.*
> *Tread cautiously.*
> *Tread curiously.*
> *Be wise to your ways.*

Out Before the Crows

This morning I am out before the crows. The sun is rising in broad stripes of deep red, pink, and purplish gray. There is a red-bellied woodpecker on the tree to my left and I hear a phoebe bird calling. I woke this morning after a persistent dream that included the line, *in the space between morning…* I dreamed this had been shared with me in the context of some kind of meaningful quote (the whole of which I remembered in the dream) and then spent the rest of the night re-dreaming this, re-discovering the quote and the message. When I woke and saw the bold exclamation of sunrise, I thought perhaps it was, *in the space between morning and doing,* but I still did not find the finished thought or message within my waking world.

As I sit on the cold stones, the crow calls start to rise out of the valley beneath me. I still don't see any, but they are rousing to morning. I follow an urge to move deeper into the woods, down the hill, past the fallen tree, and eventually over the fence. I follow an instinct to move instead of to sit and observe.

I find a well-worn forked branch partially covered with moss that looks like a skull with antlers. I muse about my relationship between *being* and *doing* and about happiness and achievement. I feel like I am no longer able to discern what I truly *want* to be doing anymore. *What is the difference, I wonder, between gentle, loving surrender, and persistence? When does one become an excuse and one become a form of self-harm?* I told Mark last night that I am going to have to try to just orient by desire and by what feels easy. Not easy as in lazy, but easy in terms of ease-full instead of painful. I do know the difference between those two feelings, but I'm not sure how to allow myself to choose between them.

I have been listening to the book *Present Over Perfect* and the author, Shauna Marie Niequist, makes the point that sometimes our greatest gift, our greatest strength, can also be the source of our greatest site of wounding in ourselves. This is how I feel this year. My relentless drive, my copious creative ability, my skill in "taking care of it" and "getting it done," is damaging me. And, to what end? To what purpose or goal? What value does this have? At the same time, I am pleased with my creations, with their impact on the world. I cannot distinguish the difference between giving up on my own unique gifts or "genius" and pushing myself to the point of destruction, exhaustion, and despair. I often feel like what I have created is too much for me, like I am too big for myself to handle any longer. I am unsure whether setting aside projects I *thought* I wanted to work on is actually just giving up during the "transition" stage of creative birthing or if it is out of some kind of fear of not being good enough. And, that if I could rise above the fears of transition, I would give birth to something absolutely wonderful. I can't decide if it is defeat from family overload and having my spirit stamped on and my passion extinguished and crushed by the demands of just living, or if it is finally pulling my life into perspective. I can't decide if it is sinking into nihilism and futility and even depression or if it is a calm Zenness of witnessing.

What I do know is that I am often unhappy and I often create this unhappiness for myself out of self-imposed expectations and demands. I sometimes feel that I can't keep up with myself, with my own relentless pace, and my own exhausting inspiration. I am not sure how to listen to what I actually *want*, how to orient by desire, but I think that is what I have left. I do know the difference between something that feels *right* and creates a sense of spaciousness, ease, and excitement and something that feels heavy, pushy, and constricting. However, I'm not sure if it is the environment around me that causes some of the things to feel heavy or if it is the projects themselves. If I didn't have other people talking to me all the time, didn't have people waiting for dinner and needing help in the bathroom, would I find the passion, purpose, drive, and excitement to finish the affirmation card project I want to create? When do I set things aside in the last stages because I'm kind of done with them on an emotional or psychic level, but with just a few more steps would create something permanent that would continue to last and be used without my continued involvement in the production of it? When does it just feel too big and too much and too heavy, because our family structure simply doesn't allow me enough *time* to actually do any of these things and instead relentlessly chops me into tinier and tinier pieces? Isn't the world full of people who become "sensible" and give up on their dreams? Is that is what I am asking of myself? To just take the easiest road, the most passive path, and to squelch out my own passion and power? *What is the difference between discernment and defeat?*

I need radical listening.

I once noted in my birth blog that there is a difference between a temporary unclenching of one's life and a permanent surrender. I continue to wonder what would happen if I just set *everything* aside and only picked back up the things I miss.

Sometimes I feel like the only things I actually *want* to do anymore are to go on small adventures in my own backyard, to walk and explore and observe what is going on around me, to write poems, to take trips and have adventures, to read, to write in my journals, to draw my oracle cards, to spend time with my goddesses and my various pretty magical things, to take pictures, and to share my little moments of inspiration and observation.

The Third Task

I do know two things: I often feel threadbare and worn and tired, oh, so tired. And that I feel joy, enchantment, delight, freedom, rapture, and happiness in the woods and when outside, anywhere, making new discoveries and observing the world.

When my final baby was born in 2014, I longed to finally just *rest*. To carve out time to just be, to sit in the chair with my baby and not feel compelled to produce, do, and speed through life. I remember holding a women's circle when he was a few weeks old. We were supposed to be making masks of one another's faces and it was important to me that I hold the event, because it was the final event in a twelve-month series—I needed to close it out, to finish it, to fulfill my commitment to myself and to the other women. As I heated up the water for tea and watched the women get comfortable, while I simultaneously nursed a baby and coached people in how to apply plaster strips to one another's faces, I longed to be the one who got to sit in the chair and drink tea with her baby, rather than being the person to get tea for others and play hostess.

At the time of this writing, that baby is now four and half years old.

I wish I didn't have to burn out so thoroughly, to feel my life force flickering so dangerously, before finally, truly, really *considering* the idea of just letting myself rest. *What would have happened if I would have just sat in the recliner and asked if someone could make me tea?*

I feel like I have been consumed.

After working for several hours in the morning, I decide to take a break and practice my daily yoga routine and have tea outside on the sunshine-blessed deck instead of in the bedroom. Making a choice like this feels like a radical act. Before I begin my yoga practice, I lie flat on my back with my arms outstretched and as I listen to the birdsong fill the air around me, I feel a sensation of my bones becoming hollow, of myself becoming hollow, of being swept through and over.

What am I ready to lay to rest? Is it the relentless striving? Forcing? Overdelivering and overperforming and overgiving?

I enjoy an extended *savasana**, with my hands resting protectively over my

---

* Lying down yoga pose.

pelvic bowl. It is time to keep some energy in.

I do an oracle card layout and write in my journals, feeling sort of emotionally flat and hollow, stilled, but in a numb sort of way, not a peaceful way. I feel like I should be figuring something out, making some kind of decision, doing something or deciding *not* to do something. As I close my journal and start to pack up my things, a vulture catches my eye again, high above me. It swoops with such ease, silently carried along by the air without flapping or trying. I wonder if this is Vulture Wisdom:

You don't have to actually move in order to be carried smoothly along by the support beneath you.

Vultures, I just learned yesterday, are the sacred bird of Hades, Lord of the Underworld and mate of Persephone, whether by choice or by force. They have no voicebox and do not make noise. I am fascinated by vultures, especially the way they glide with such grace across the sky. They are so often overlooked as "gross" or treated as a bad omen, but I look at them with appreciation for how much they take care of, clean up, make tidy once more. They consume flesh, but they do not kill. They come to do the work that others shy away from. They waste nothing. They digest what is unwanted and leave a cleaner world. They are vigilant, graceful and observant: quiet watchers of the skies. When I watch them fly, I feel like I, too, somehow know what it feels like to soar across the clouds, like a speed skater on air, buoyed with the knowing that I am carried capably by support beneath me. I wonder what might happen for me with more opportunity for silence, less of an urge to share, or communicate, but perhaps rather bearing quiet witness from high above, knowing I will not fall.

The third task
is to learn
how to rest.

Dancing with Limitation

This morning the woods are quiet and the sky is once again a gray bowl hanging heavily over the landscape. I see one crow, though I hear several more, and one quiet robin. A mourning dove calls in the distance.

I am thinking about boundaries, limits, shoring up my banks, letting things go to drift on the breeze, about how to coast with life instead of how to wrestle it into my control. After my radical rest on the deck in the sunshine yesterday, I've decided that the time has come to truly set some limits on our work time, hours, and devotion.

As I listen to the crows in the woods, I realize that this will be the task, or initiation of Air for me: *cleansing and releasing.* While I'm not finished learning from Air, not by a long shot, I can sense the tasks and lessons of the other elements in the future:

> *Air is for cleansing.*
> *Earth is for strengthening.*
> *Water is for healing.*
> *Fire is for rekindling, reigniting.*

This is how I will rebuild my life and live my story.

This is how I will stand up for myself. This is how I will restore my soul. I will not wait for later or the "right time." There is only *this time* and I am ready to live in it.

I am tired of living my *real life* only in snatches or in stolen moments. *What if I recognize that all of my life is my real life?* I am responsible, or capable, of bringing it into alignment with my values and priorities, instead of waiting for the scraps of "extra time" that too-rarely come.

I read a section in Day Schildkret's book *Morning Altars* about limitation.

> *I have a limited conception of limitation. It makes me feel defeated and like I've failed to accept limits. What if limitation is a necessary facet of depth of living and creative existence?*

He then quotes Anne Bogart as writing:

> *Limits are a necessary partner in the creative act as well as in the crafting of a successful life. What matters is the ability to look around and accurately recognize what is working for you and what is working against you, adjusting to the realities of the situation and mining the potential of the limits with invention and energy.*

I begin to wonder…

How might I dance with limitation and view it as fuel for wholeness, instead of grounds for despair? Might it even be possible to love my limits, learn from them, lean into them?

> *May I risk stretching out*
> *trembling fingers,*
> *may I risk the cracking open,*
> *may I risk eating the seeds of truth.*
> *May I risk arriving*
> *at the gates of the Underworld,*
> *shivering and naked,*
> *flowers in my hands.*

Passion and Purpose

I have trouble sleeping and wake at 4 a.m. to lie there restless and disturbed, wondering if I really even want to continue working in this way. Holding regular women's circles, it seems, is another commitment that I can no longer discern if it is based in actual desire or in obligation. I'm noticing a seven-year cycle of passion and purpose in my life, where I am wholeheartedly invested in something for seven years, maybe even overly invested, and then it starts to feel like a burden and I have to let it go, even becoming desperate to let it go. *Is this my fault for being "too passionate" about life in general? Do I set myself up for burnout simply with the way I approach my tasks and interests with total commitment and excessive giving to make whatever it is the best it can be…then, wear myself out, feel unappreciated, reach a breaking point, and drive myself to the point where the only door left is out, to quit?*

I was ordained as a priestess exactly seven years ago, though I held circles and ceremonies for many years before I felt worthy of claiming the mantle of priestess. I taught college classes for, you guessed it, seven years. I lost my heart for birth education after seven years also, but forced myself to continue for ten years and the same with La Leche League, where I served as a volunteer breastfeeding peer counselor for ten years. After pouring myself into something, I find the appetite I feel from others to consume me is never-ending and I have to pull back in order, it feels, to preserve my own life force. As I lie there sleeplessly, I review the amount of times I've turned my kids away because I'm helping someone else who "needs me," but who evaporates from my life as soon as I set boundaries on my giving or my availability.

I call upon Vulture as my brain spins these ruts sleeplessly and with increasing agitation and with a sensation of fruitlessness and despair.

Make me a hollow bone, I call, *sweep me clean.*

Digest this ugly waste and clear the landscape of my life so that new things may flourish.

Make me a hollow bone. Sweep me clean. Pick me over.

Turn me inside out and scour my bones.

It feels risky and scary to call upon Vulture in this way.

What if I'm making a mistake?

What if I don't really want a clean start?

What if I don't want my bones chewed on?

What I *do* need is that which is decaying within me to be rooted out and released. I need perspective, clarity of vision, and the opportunity to swoop over my life with a broad gaze determined to clear out that which is finished.

I feel a coolness sweep through my body, my hands relax, and I sleep.

One of my fears in inviting myself to be stripped bare is worrying I will lose something of my essential self. Something that makes me so *me*, my truest gift and offering.

What if I find out that everything I have been doing is just to prove my worthiness?

What if I am not worthy?

At the same time, what if I uncover something that has actually been lost, buried under years of doing and offering and pleasing? What if my essential self is exactly what will be revealed and I will discover a core of worthiness that has been obscured by years of a service-equals-worth behavior and conditioning?

What if my wholeness is right there, waiting to be reborn?

The Fourth Task

I sit on the cold stones this morning, under a gray sky on this, the first day of spring. Raindrops patter down around me. I don't see or hear the crows and the woods are relatively quiet, other than the gentle sound of raindrops. I recognize that I am aware of a core of fiery resolve within me and rather than feel like it is being extinguished, it feels like it is being strengthened.

It is the first day of spring and another day of homeschool co-op. When I go to the urban lake between classes, I find a curved root that reminds me of a curled-up woman and I put a goddess figurine inside for a photo. As I do so, a poem from Persephone suddenly rises up within me, I hear the first lines as if they have been waiting for me to trip over them, to pick them up.

> *I have slumbered*
> *in shadowed places*
> *not knowing the surface*
> *from the shore.*

I found this poem, I feel, in these tangles of roots that look like the ruins of lost cities. I look up suddenly and, no joke, a lone vulture is circling in the air.

I feel called to move onward, further along the bank of the lake, to a section I have not visited before. As I walk more lines for the poem rise up to meet me. Persephone is speaking as if she is responding to my footsteps.

> *I have learned what it means to*
> *rise soft-bellied from the deep*
> *shards of darkness clinging*
> *to my thighs,*
> *my lips stained berry-red*
> *with truth and desire,*
> *my heart still capable*
> *of shedding flowers*
> *and drops of hope*
> *on hungry plains*
> *and stark forests*

A cardinal sings from a nearby oak as I approach a small thicket of thin trees, branches wound together forming a tunnel with a path through it. I would have to crawl to move through the tunnel, so I think it is made by animals, not humans. I crouch down in the thicket and two mourning doves rise up to settle on different branches in front of me. I take some pictures as a small shaft of sunlight begins to emerge from the gray sky.

> *while mourning doves*
> *rise from secret thickets,*
> *and the yearning*
> *in my bones*
> *pulls me to both rise*
> *and sink.*

I return to the knobbed tiny root city shoreline, and sit with my back against one, legs stretched out on damp ground littered with goose droppings. The sun continues to make a slender path of light across the water and I finish my poem, feeling awed, humbled, and grateful at being right here at this moment to discover it, to pick it up, to let it flow through my fingers. It is as if Persephone has suddenly risen up in front of my eyes, ready for the springtime. I hear her voice move through me as if she's gently cast a thread of connection through time and space to settle on me, as if I'm drawing the words from her directly through this shimmering, delicate thread.

Six months from this moment I learn that the tiny root cities, the curled root woman, and the ferny evergreen trees are cypress trees and not a variety of cedar as I first assumed. Cypress is a classic tree of Greek landscapes and, in fact, is the tree sacred to Hades and a symbol of the Underworld.

> *There is sunrise passion*
> *in my eyes,*
> *a pulse of longing in*
> *my center,*
> *a blush of firelight*
> *streaked across my skin,*
> *where sunshine*
> *meets shadow*
> *again*
> *and again.*

When I return to the co-op building I feel altered, aware of the fiery core of resolve within my chest, but also tasting the sensation of what it feels like to rise from the deep, shards of darkness clinging to my thighs, and my lips stained berry-red with truth and desire.

At home, I set up the simplest of altars—an herbed candle and two small goddesses, a spring maiden and her purple magic mother. We circle in the sunset-moonrise on the deck, anointing one another's heads with scented oil floating with lavender buds. My four-year-old anoints my head, me kneeling, laughing on the deck as he tips it carefully and seriously onto my forehead. My teenage sons anoint each other's, touching me with the stab of poignancy and gratitude that they are here with me, willing to dab fragrant, flower-laden oil onto one another's faces as they both deepen into manhood before my eyes. We burn an herb bundle and waft the sacred smoke around one another's bodies, my eight-year-old daughter sweeping the burning bundle around my husband, stretching her arm up high to bless his heart and head. We hold small pinches of wildflower seeds in our hands and share seasonal intentions with one another, then move to the front of the house singing the whole time as we scatter the seeds of our promises into the flower box. We return to the deck, still singing, then join hands around our candle, offering a simple prayer and then howling at the moon.

This has been very simple ritual, largely spontaneous, based on the tools and mood at hand and it feels perfect. I remember how I used to put so much effort into set up and planning and then be bothered when the mood or energy of what I was trying to create was "destroyed" by the unpredictability of children and how they often lack of patience with standing in a circle for a long time musing about universal truths. It is interesting to witness how the less effort I put into planning the ceremony in advance, the more beautiful and meaningful the actual rituals I hold for my family have become: authentic to *our* family in this time and place, not scripted for the consumption or benefit of others. I wonder if my Red Tent would feel the same if I eased up completely, if I just let it emerge naturally, would it then become even richer, deeper, and more tender?

As I blow out my candle, I blow a kiss to the moon and say, *Thank you.*

The spirit and energy of our simple, unscripted, naturally evolving ritual lingers in the air with the touch of magic and love. My husband carries the burning herbs through all the rooms of our house and to the doors and porches as well, letting the smoke waft into hidden corners and bringing a sensation of vitality, renewal, and change to the stale winter air. The smell of the smoke lingers too and along with my core of resolve, I feel the rising energy of anticipation, excitement, and joy.

This is real magic.

This ceremony to welcome spring brings to mind our Winter Solstice three months back, when we walked our traditional candlelit Solstice spiral together under a rising full moon. During the ritual, I breathed a seed dream promise of balance into a small amethyst sphere pendant, which I put around my neck, promising not to take it off until it separated of its own accord, knowing then my seed dream would be realized. The ritual theory behind a seed dream pendant is that it will incubate through Imbolc and then start to gradually push through towards the light of the Spring Equinox. As I muse about family and work, I put my fingers up to my throat to touch my pendant, this seed dream promise...it gently separates and falls away into my hand.

> *The fourth task*
> *is to keep your promises*
> *to yourself.*

Persephone's Lessons

This morning as I sit on the rocks in the early morning sunshine I continue to reflect on Persephone and what I can learn from her story. This is her season and her story is one of rebirth and renewal, as well as having given up much of her old identity, shedding layers of herself on her descent into the Underworld. She is actually the perfect goddess for my journey of renewal, cleansing, and rebirth with Air.

As I think this, the sky suddenly darkens, completely hiding the sun — it is so abrupt that it startles me and then quickly a shaft of sunlight emerges again, shining directly where I sit. I close my eyes and tilt my face to the sun, feeling the warmth and seeing the dancing sparkles of light under my eyelids. This feels like Persephone too, in the meeting of sunlight and shadow across my skin. The breeze dances around, caressing my body and lifting my hair, sweeping along my spine, and curving around my shoulders.

I remember how at our Red Tent retreat this past fall, my message from a guided meditation was that I was ready to shed the sensation of feeling forced. At our spring retreat, the message was: *I am free to choose.* I turn to go inside, saying thank you as I do so, when I hear:

You should leave an offering in return.

I pluck out two strands of my hair, hold them aloft and let the breeze catch them and carry them away.

In the late afternoon I make the radical choice to go outside in the middle of working and just lie on my back in the sunshine. It is shocking how radical this feels, even though I lose nothing, work-wise, in terms of doing it and only gain mental health and spiritual well-being.

I wanted to take my books and journals and my colored pens too, but I am not that radical yet! I am still thinking about Persephone, what she teaches about descent and rebirth, renewal and return. I reach out to her with my mind, starting to form a prayer, a pleading, a request for learning…*Persephone*…I call. A shadow crosses my closed eyelids, I open them to see a lone vulture coast by.

Persephone,
please walk with me.
May I be brave enough
to orient my life by desire.
May I choose freely
with an understanding
of sovereignty.
May I choose boldly
and without regret.
May I release myself
from expectation, should,
and obligation.
May I trust desire and longing
as my guides.

Otherworldly Journeys are
Most Definitely Afoot

I am in the woods at sunrise, my bottom chilling on cold stones, ready to make a promise, to invite next steps and next processes. There are crows calling all around me and the back-and-forth greetings of two mourning doves rising and falling. I stretch out my awareness to Persephone, inviting the possibility of walking on her path. I speak a combination of prayer and invocation, invitation and longing. Two crows busily fly by on their morning route.

> *I open to your presence*
> *I am open to your power*
> *I am open to your possibility*
> *I am open to your path.*
> *I am making a promise now*
> *to split my life open*
> *before your eyes*
> *and choose*
> *which seeds to eat*
> *which to plant*
> *and which to cast back*
> *into the Underworld…*

As I speak these words, I hear the distinctive and completely unexpected call of a barred owl in the woods. While I hear this owl at night sometimes, I have never once heard it in the morning. It literally feels like I have been answered by Persephone herself and I feel a profound sense of gratitude at receiving such a clear reply.

I have a strong and certain sensation that this is the next phase. Persephone arrived in my awareness in the windy whispers at an urban lake on the first day of spring, and we will walk together, work together for at least three months, for a complete season. I will need to offer her something in return, and then this stage of my soul rebuilding will be complete and I will move into another phase of this journey of restoration into wholeness. I put on a garnet bracelet as a symbol of my commitment and know that when it falls off or breaks, it will indicate this part of my work is done. I sit with my eyes closed in the rising sun, visualizing

Persephone walking towards me.

> *Persephone,*
> *please walk with me.*
> *Please grant me fortitude of spirit,*
> *clarity of mind,*
> *and steadfastness of heart.*
> *Please encourage me,*
> *please inspire me,*
> *please guide me into freedom,*
> *purpose,*
> *and passion.*

I open my hands on my lap and my right hand fills with warmth, despite the cold morning air, as if I have been taken by the hand. My palm feels glowing, strong, and almost hot. I touch it gently to my forehead, my eyes, my throat, my heart, my belly, and my legs.

My invitation has been accepted.

I again offer two strands of my hair into the light breeze and follow the mossy path back home.

When I get back inside, I am startled to see that more than forty-five minutes have passed since I left the house, even though it feels like it has been only fifteen.

Otherworldly journeys and initiations are definitely afoot, I say to Mark with laughter in my voice.

He is mired down in tax preparation for the rest of the day, so we don't get to go for our late afternoon walk. I go out with our two youngest children instead, to explore the woods behind the house. We walk for a long way, down in the ravine behind our house, where we climb on moss-strewn stones and listen to the gentle trickle of water falling. While the walk is nice overall, I spent more of today than I would like feeling overextended, impatient, and full of other people's voices, my journals and oracle cards lying unexplored on the floor of the living room, while I try to fulfill the endless needs of these small people, who never seem to quite feel that I'm enough. I think about Persephone as Daughter and of the expectations we hold of our children and that they hold of us.

Later, I drive my daughter to a sleepover at her friend's house. We see eleven vultures circling the road and I tell the kids, *these are my friends now. We're getting to know each other.* After dropping off Alaina, I go to the grocery store with my youngest son and we pick out a bouquet of red carnations for our altar. I also buy a glass jar full of glistening red pomegranate juice.

Being Responsible

I wake up this morning realizing it absolutely makes sense to start with Persephone. What better guide for an Underworld journey of rebuilding a soul? That is the very stuff of her story and now it is part of mine. I must travel below, excavate the shards, the wreckage, and rise above the surface again. I must find the seeds of my life and examine them. Seeds need to be nourished in dark places in order to grow, yes, *but what if what I've planted isn't what I actually want anymore?*

What have I put my heart into growing that I no longer need?

What have I let wither and decay?

I have always had an intense quality about me. I have always thought deeply, taken things seriously, and been committed to my direction in life. At some point, though, I've lost sight of anything but the drive, the push, the fervor to get more and more and more done. I remember walking to the mailbox with Mark at least twelve years ago and saying, *I really don't want people to say after I die: 'Well, she sure got a lot done, but she never really had any fun.'* And here I am at forty, with fun reserved only for small slices and stolen moments.

I try to remember when I learned that I could please people and be approved of for getting things done. *Be responsible. Take care of it. Fulfill your commitments. Meet your obligations. Excel in All Things.* Is that hardwired in me? Feeling this compulsion to get things done, to do it all, to achieve, to be good, to be worthy. There is nothing *wrong* with honoring your commitments, true, but when commitments are made out of a misplaced desire to prove yourself worthy of *being*, there *is* something wrong.

Several weeks ago, I was asked for help from a friend and as I tried to fit in a reply, I realized my own life is too close a breaking point, too taut and strained to do One. More. Thing. In the rush to get the kids ready for co-op, to pack my class supplies, to hold my threadbare soul together, I didn't answer her message requesting my aid. A line from Mary Oliver kept replaying in my brain:

Determined to save the only life you can save: your own.

There is a part of me that has been "saving lives" for others for decades, while the pool of resources reserved for my own inner life shrinks smaller and smaller and I feel more and more thirsty for myself.

It is perhaps in college that my compulsion to succeed, to prove and prove again, truly takes root almost like a sickness. I am fifteen and half when I start college. I finished my homeschool high school curriculum in fourteen months instead of four years and it seems like college is the next logical choice. *Is this where the need to prove I am worthy begins? Or, were the seeds planted earlier?* I'm not sure, but it definitely provided cultivation and nourishment of this compulsion. Since my earliest memories, I have always liked to win, I have always liked to be in charge, I have always liked to lead. I was always the teacher, the mom, the boss, when I played make-believe scenarios as a child with my friends. I have always had a "strong personality" and a tendency towards being bossy, controlling, and taking the lead. These are not bad qualities, but when nourished in a hot house of pressure and performance, they can become overgrown, untended, and wild, crowding out all else that might wish to grow. Now, I am tired. I want to lay down some, or all, of this caretaking and giving and controlling and leading and sit in the woods. And I want to do this by choice, by intention, not by being forced into it by poor health or mental illness.

The Cauldron

Each year in the summer, I feel sped up to the point of collapse, taking on more and more and more until I am ready to fall apart. Each year, I say to Mark, *this pace is not sustainable. If I keep going like this, something bad will happen to me.*

And then I keep going.

This year, I refuse to wait until July to say no. Just in time to collapse into Cauldron Month.

I have honored what I call a "Cauldron Month" for myself each August, after a meditation in which I experienced a powerful vision of the Cauldron rune emblazoned on the floor of my tiny temple building. It is always a very powerful time and I crave the opportunity to do it each year.

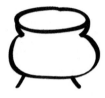

The Cauldron in the Womanrunes oracle system is a rune of alchemy and change, but also of containment and contemplation—a marrying of what might seem like opposites, but that which really co-exist. The Cauldron asks us what we're cooking, but it also offers boundaries, containment, and a safe space in which to stew up our truest magic. "Taking it all to the cauldron" means a time in which to let it all bubble and brew and stew and percolate. I pull my energy inward to let myself listen and be and to see what wants to emerge.

Last year, even though I took two whole months in the Cauldron, the pace continued to accelerate through the Yuletide season and though I experienced a blessed reprieve at the beach in January, upon returning home the pace immediately reached July-level-speed even though it was only February. The thoughts recur: *I can't keep going like this. The pace is not sustainable. If I keep going this way, something bad will happen to me.* I spent February and early March almost constantly at the edge of tears, feeling brittle and worn thin with strain.

In many ways, this year is feeling like a Cauldron Year for me, a time to listen, to steep, to watch, to learn, and to wait.

I will rebuild my soul.

Even if that means saying no to almost everything else in the process. Project ideas, book ideas, class ideas, product ideas, all can be laid to rest, or at least set aside for an undetermined length of time.

I often find myself thinking that if I can create the amount of magic that I do around the edges, margins, and scraps of my life, *what might I create with a day, a week, a month, a year if I move devotion to experiencing into the center of my life instead of on the periphery?*

I can have fun. I can laugh in the sunshine and take long walks through forgotten thickets on moss-laden stones.

The Fifth Task

This morning, I sit on the rocks holding one of my red carnations as an offering for Persephone. I press it to my lips, feeling the way the petals part. I think about taking a picture of the carnation, the blood red richness of its petals. But then I don't.

Some things are not meant to be shared.

I am realizing this slowly. Sometimes you must hold the tender parts of yourself in secret places, in the planes of life and living, the shafts of sunlight, and the drifts of shadow, the trickles of wonder and the rivers of wondering.

I kiss the red carnation one more time and say, *I brought this for you.*

Right as I lay it on the rocks, a silent crow swoops across my line of vision, tracing the tree-lined horizon and away over the roof of my house.

I think about the different versions of Persephone's tale, some involving free will and active choice and others about force.

Nothing forced.

I will learn from Persephone and the elements.

Later in the day I am teaching a writing class for teenagers and we are using letter stamps to create short messages in our class art journals. They encourage me to stamp something I keep telling them during class: *no forcing.* This feels in some ways, like the motto for my writing class, but also perhaps like a title for a new book of poems. *No forcing.* Just living and looking. *What will we see if we stop trying to make something happen?* I take a photo of my stamped journal page by the lakeside, two geese in the foreground. Right as I click the button for the photo, one goose stretches its wings open to full width. It doesn't fly away, but folds them back in against its body, after this good stretch.

As I walk back to the parking lot, I hear the cry of a hawk in the gray sky high above me. I feel as if the lake and I now share a secret—what it feels like to stand in the wind and rain together, under a wide sky.

The fifth task is
no forcing.

Pain and Growth

I wake this morning from a dream in which I am pursued by a man and a dog. I feel heavy and weary, weighed down by my never-ending to-do list. I feel like curling inward on myself, because I am tired. So tired. I don't want to serve as "fuel" for anyone else anymore. I am done. Burned out, fried, used up. I've lost my "help others" instinct which mutated into "please others" which mutated into "fuel others"...and I'm *out*. Out of steam. Out of drive. Out of enthusiasm. My fire has dimmed to embers and I just want to pull inside and away and see if I can keep my own coals burning, close to my heart, fueling only myself. My "make a difference" drive has fueled and pushed me for decades and now I'm exhausted. *Was it ever really about making a difference or just about trying to be worthwhile?* I feel as if I've finally let myself be extinguished. I feel drained of reserves. I feel private and pulled in. Incubating and composting.

A quote comes into my email at just the right moment:

Spring does not simply blow upon the warming air like blossom kisses. Spring is as much a time of pain as of growth. Imagine the egg, the bulb, the bud. All begin contained—all potential, endless promise. There is quiet dignity in such presence...

But when growth begins, things break. Shells and bud casings, those intact perfections, fall away. What is revealed is unprotected tenderness...growth may be exhilarating, but it is never easy.

— **Patricia Monaghan**, *Seasons of the Witch:*
Poetry and Songs to the Goddess

Yes. I feel this pain and this growth. Something is cracking and falling away.

> *let me split my life open*
> *gaze at the red pomegranate seeds within*
> *and eat*
> *knowing that some part of me*
> *will remain*
> *in the Underworld forever.*

Persephone Ritual

I am alone for the first time in a week and the house is blissfully silent. I guard the silence, the need to curl inward, rather than rushing to get my work done.

This day is a precious gift.

So too, is examining my soul fragments. So too, retrieving myself from where I have wandered, listening to and learning from my own heart, which seems to only be heard when there is enough space for whispers.

It is time for dedication.

It is time to devote myself to making myself whole once more. It is time for devotion to this path of unfolding discovery and change. I feel the call coiled within me, alive and pulsing. I must bring this commitment I am making into visible form, I must dedicate myself to this work, to this listening, to this learning.

I prepare for a Persephone ritual, packing a basket with my vulture feather, pomegranate juice, a red carnation, a candle, my white shawl, my goddess figurines, and a bar of chocolate. I step through the woods and onto the rocks that have borne witness to so many other dedications and promises, to my ordination as a priestess, to my tears and my laughter, to the births of books and the blessing of new children, to my deep love, and to my deep sorrow. I have come to offer a promise of renewal and prayer of homecoming for my soul as well as a ritual of offering and initiation. I am promising at least the next three months to listen, to learn, to study—Air and Persephone, the goddess and the element.

I pour pomegranate juice into a cut glass dish as a symbol of choosing—choosing with full consciousness and intention. I also offer it as a symbol of my own blood, my *life force*, my ability to choose freely and courageously, to set aside the sensation of force and to accept the mantle of choice. A symbol of my commitment to the renewal of my body and soul and to walking this path with Persephone into the Underworld, preparing to emerge, rebirthed into my own wholeness and capacity. A reminder that I must fuel myself, fuel my soul, before I fuel anything else. I must receive nourishment. I must accept nourishment. I must be open to nourishment. I must actively choose to take it in.

After pouring a little onto the leaves and stones, I drink the ruby red juice, drawing it into me.

My choice is to be an active initiator of my own life and path. When I feel the sensation of 'no' rising up within me, I have a responsibility to listen to it, to honor it, and to set limits on what I am able to provide. I feel the core of fiery resolve within me once more and I can trust it. I must trust it.

I offer the flower next. May it be a symbol of my own tenderness, the blossoming of what I hold and give and share and offer and nourish. May these offerings be conscious and intentional, may they be freely offered from a place of growth, health, stability, and love.

The candle is a symbol of my own flame, which feels like it is flickering, but which will be needed to guide me through darkness. I am asking for help in nourishing my flame, my core of fiery resolve. *Please, please help me keep it from fading, please help me to tend it and kindle it anew.*

My white shawl is a symbol of initiation and dedication, but it is also a symbol of renewal and protection that will drape around me as a reminder that it is okay to cocoon, to draw inward, to be still, to be silent, to incubate and renew, to hold myself tenderly and inwardly without guilt.

The last element of my ritual is the vulture feather, gracefully and unexpectedly gifted, gracefully and unexpectedly received. I use it as a feather wand, sweeping it around my arms and legs and head and belly. Just as a vulture knows how to clean up, clear out, digest, and expel that which is not needed any longer, I, too, can trust this discernment in myself.

It is time to shed these patterns of thought that no longer work for me about my life, my work, my business. It is time to release them, to set them free in these currents of air, trusting that life is buoyant enough to carry me without wrestling, struggling, and controlling, but letting myself coast on the ample support beneath me and around me and through me.

> *I look up and learn from the birds.*
> *I open my hands to be caressed by the air.*
> *I open my heart to excavate the red seeds within.*
> *May I accept nourishment.*
> *May I be alert for,*
> *open to,*
> *and accepting of*
> *the hand of Persephone in my own*
> *as we journey together*
> *through the Underworld*
> *back up into the sunshine*
> *renewed and whole*
> *having been courageous enough*

to leave something of ourselves behind
to cast off that which is unnecessary
and sometimes
that which is painful
and sometimes
that which is unwanted.

Cast it off, lay it down, let it drift, and then rise soft-bellied from the deep.

Today is a fresh beginning. A new start. A cleansing. An initiation. A promise. But, also, it is only a beginning. A step on the path, but a beginning step, not a completion. It is a release, a renewal, and a promise to learn, to change.

May I have the courage to change.

Please.

I lay the feather down and lie back on the cold stones, gazing up at the dark fingers of the tree branches against the gray sky.

I am offering myself up to change.
I am offering myself up to be renewed.
I am offering myself up to be rebuilt.
I am offering myself up to listen and learn.
I am offering myself up to be nourished and restored.
I will trust in the signs and signals I am given.
I will tend to and nourish my relationships with myself
and my family as primary, rather than with the remaining
scraps of myself after the rest has been given away.
I have wanted this for a long time.
Please receive my dedication, my offerings, my
commitment, my small human self, with all her
wishes and longings and scars and triumphs.
It is all that I have.

I sit back up. I anoint myself with oil to seal my promises and eat my chocolate to ground myself. I will carry my talismans and my commitment and focus through the next part of the year. I will carefully observe what I learn, what I need, and what I know I need to do. At the same time, may there be light and joy and delight in my heart, beneath my feet, and in my arms. While this Underworld journey of recovery and reclamation on which I embark may be dark and heavy, there is joyful promise here too: the delight of renewal and rebirth. I will fling my arms open to the sunshine and the blossoming, to that which will help me to grow and be whole.

I'm ready to learn.

I blow out the candle, offering my thanks and blessing that the ritual is complete. The wind swirls and rises around me.

There is silence for a moment.

And then I see the two hawks again, further away above the field.

This feels like enough. An acceptance of my offering.

But then a silent shadow crosses above my head, and two vultures soar past me on wings of ease.

The next morning my four-year-old asks to join me in the woods to go exploring. I feel a bit cramped and resistant to relinquishing my solitude, but then I soften into it. This small person with blonde hair and such an eager face, just wanting to be with me. He practices his jumping from stone to stone, exclaiming at his own prowess. He asks me, *Mom, why are you hugging me so much?*

Because, my boy, I tell him, *you are glowing.*

We discover that my offering of pomegranate juice has been accepted, cut glass bowl empty and gleaming in the sunlight as if it has been washed. We sit in the sun for a moment, my eyelashes sun-spangled, the canes of wild raspberries glimmering with purple shadow.

When we return inside, we toast one another with pottery cups of pomegranate juice, celebrating our small adventure. *You're my best mama in the whole world,* he says, *and you still have one tiny boy who loves you.* He curls on my lap as small as possible, still fitting there, blond head beneath my chin, legs tucked up against his chest.

What is at the Center of your Life?

I wake to a gray morning with the pulse of pain behind my eyes and feeling a little sick. This is a familiar aftermath of communication fatigue and also often a symptom of having taught or held circle the night before. Sometimes I jokingly call them "priestess headaches," but indeed, they're not a joke, but a very real sign from my body that I've moved a lot of energy through me and have perhaps depleted something of my own core in the process.

I head for the woods immediately, gray stones, green moss, gray sky.

What is at the center of your life?

This question pulses in my chest this morning. I lay my hand on the thin, warm skin of my chest at the base of my throat.

What is at the center of my life?

It starts to rain. Small droplets at first and then bigger and bigger, thrumming on the slick surface of my down jacket. I pull up the hood and sit in my cocoon, feeling cut off from the sharp sensory input I usually experience here, but also withdrawn and safe.

What is at the center?

I cast my mind out to Persephone. *Did she feel a core of fiery resolve within her as she set off into the Underworld, or was she shaken, frightened, and uncertain? Was it love that called her to dive beneath or was it fear? Was it choice or force?* I realize that regardless of which brought her below, it was the core of fiery resolve that brought her to the surface again. I can lean into this. This sensation. This core. This determination. It can guide my next steps.

I have to refuel. I must listen.

What do I trust? Can I hear the "deeper river"? What is at the center of my living truth?

I need time. Always time. More time. And silence.

There is something here. Something thrumming below the surface of everyday reality. I want to pay attention. I want to attune to this rhythm. I want to hear and be heard. I want to watch. I want to learn. I want more than snatches and whispers and glimmers and moments, I want to throw myself into this ensouled and enchanting world. I want to be in dialog with myself, with my heart, with my soul, but also with the Goddess, She Who Holds the Whole, She Who Weaves the All, without having to wait for stolen moments and scraps of time.

When I started on a goddess path, I had a craving for spiritual contact, for an awareness of the Goddess as a living reality, a living presence on (and in) this earth and world. I glimpsed her clearly at times, woven through my days, but it wasn't until I'd spent at least seven years of dedicated, regular study, practices, trainings, education, and classes that my awareness changed to a constant thread of connection with her. It is always there. I can extend my awareness and *always* feel it. I call this "life in the palm of her hand" and awareness of that truth is what softened my drive to "prove" her to anyone else. I don't need to prove it, when I inhabit her world.

My issue now becomes remembering to stretch out to touch the thread of connection *even when life is stressful and the house is chaotic.* Even when I have "too much to do" and feel scattered, fragmented, and overwhelmed. That is when I need to remember to *connect anyway.* I have spent years feeling like I use up something of myself, give away parts of my own soul, my own life force, in service to others. I *have* to remember, as they taught me in reiki training, that the energy you draw up in service to others can be sourced from the support *around you,* it doesn't have to be drawn from, or out of, your own core. Drawing from your own core instead of from the whole is how you become depleted. I feel like I have a high reserve of energy, I feel like I have a strong core, I feel like I have a resourceful, connected soul. And I feel like I have spent years tapping *that* energy, the energy within me, to fuel other people's journeys and experiences.

I need to rebuild my boundaries as I rebuild my soul.

When I return indoors, I page through my art journal from the last eight weeks. I see in the place where I have drawn out my questions of the year that I have written:

What is at the center of your living truth?

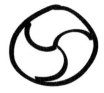

I choose my Womanrunes card of the day and receive The Wheel. I have learned with practice that the best way to draw this rune is to start at the center and then make the spokes coming outward from a central dot. I used to try to draw the lines to meet in the center, without having a center dot and in this way one segment was always off kilter. When you start from the center, the Wheel is balanced.

The connection strikes me suddenly.

You must begin from the center and expand from there.

If you start at the outside of the "wheel" of your life and then try to add spokes to your wheel, you won't get it "right"—there will be unevenness, imbalance, and things that don't work. If you start from the center, you can consciously, intentionally, draw out from the center and expand.

Have I been living from the center of my own life, or have I been living from the spokes? Have I been trying to connect spokes without a firm center to anchor them? I've observed in my group work, women's circle work, and community building that a community, a group, needs a strong "center-holder" to keep the group organized. A healthy group also needs many other things, but without a center-holder, the group will collapse in on itself. Composing a personal life is the same—we each must hold our center and *then*, only then, radiate outward into the other aspects of our lives.

The Sixth Task

Mark and I go for a walk on our gravel road this evening. When we first step outside, there is a fallen tree branch on our electric box. When we step over nearer to see, a bird suddenly swoops up, it hangs in a gust of air above the field, ragged wings extended like a kite, seeming to be caught, immobile in the sharp thrust of air. I think at first it is our hawk friend and my heart swells, but it is actually a vulture. We watch it break from the current of air and continue to coast away over the horizon.

The wind is ferocious and there is no sunset. The ground is littered with fragments of cedar and small oak branches. At one point the wind howls so deeply, that we look up at the swaying trees above us and feel a small frisson of fear pass through us.

We are vulnerably human in a big world.

> *The sixth task*
> *is to show up*
> *for everything.*

Life is Not a Problem to be Solved

Work is accelerated and relentless today as we prepare to shut up shop and take our family away on vacation. I feel frustrated with myself, like I'm supposed to be learning more, doing better, *being* better. I keep feeling an insistent tug to go back outside and just stand for a few minutes, but I ignore the impulse and keep on working. I start reflecting as I work on how often I've chided myself for not "figuring it all out." I think I've spent the majority of my adult life thinking there is a "right answer" and when I *finally* figure it out things will be easy, I will be "good enough," everything will be figured out and settled. If I "fail" to figure it out, it means I'm a hypocrite who has nothing of value to offer or teach. Right?!

A knowing arises in me: *your self is not an enemy and you are not a problem to be solved.* I do, in fact, trust my self, just as I trust my hands, my senses, and my lungs. The self is not an enemy or a problem, but is actually a healthy, whole part of being a living, breathing creature on this earth. *If you start from the perspective that the self is not a problem to be solved, any conflict softens and dissolves.*

If you cannot trust your self, what can you trust? Perhaps it is just that the wind will carry you, where you need to go, that the trees will sway, that the rocks will be cold, that the rain will come and go.

I take a few minutes time out and lie on the floor, with my arms outstretched. I dab some rose anointing oil on my neck and chest. I sit with my hand on my belly:

Persephone, please walk with me.

I move my hand to my chest and sit in stillness for a few minutes.

It clicks. This is Persephone's teaching. Life is cyclical. Once she has descended to the Underworld and she has made her way along its terrain, she resurfaces. But she does not stay risen permanently, she descends again. And rises again. And descends again. This is the work of human living too. Peaks and valleys. Highs and lows. Ebbs and flows. Tidal rhythm. Seasonal rhythm. Life rhythm. Hormonal rhythm.

We are surrounded by cycles, we are surrounded by ever-changing landscapes, feelings, bodies, and other people. The tides come and the tides go. The sun rises and the sun sets. The rain falls and the sun shines. There simply is no permanent *figured out*. It is okay for me to feel content and centered one day and frazzled and overloaded another. I'd like to shift the balance between those two, of course, but the reality of what Jennifer Louden terms a "human-sized life" is that sometimes life is frazzling, sometimes there is too much to do in any one day. What I'm seeking to shift is the percentage of my days I spend in frazzled mode, to consciously choose and mindfully attend to my rhythms, so that my capacity to tend to my soul, listen to my heart and refuel my spirit is enhanced, rather than depleted, but not to expect that after a series of lessons or tasks that my work is then *done*. Complete. Forever. No, if there is anything the earth teaches, that Persephone teaches, it is that the cycle then begins anew.

This work is not easy.

It is still worth it.

I realize now why I have never been called to walk with Persephone before. She seems too tender, too vulnerable, too not "in control" of her own destiny. It is more comforting and reassuring to work with a powerful goddess, one who can get it all figured out. But this is actually exactly *why* Persephone now, because she has been vulnerable, she has been afraid, she has been unwilling. She has journeyed into the Underworld and returned. She has faced fear and doubt and confusion and loss and grief. She has sunk and she has risen. What better partner to explore this terrain with, this landscape of the forgotten, the unwanted, the discarded, the ignored, the silenced, the voiceless, the crying out from within? This is Persephone's terrain, her landscape, her area of expertise, her realm, and her area of power.

> *If life is not a problem,*
> *to be solved,*
> *but an experience to*
> *be lived,*
> *might you become aware*
> *of the soft breath*
> *in your belly*
> *the pull of need*
> *in your back*
> *the dawning realization*
> *that there is nothing to do*
> *and nothing to prove*
> *and you are safe*
> *in being on this earth.*
> *It is okay to be,*

to watch,
to know and not know.
To be curious.
To soften into longing
and feel it spread
across your shoulders
and into the rise and fall
of your chest.
Where are you going?
Here.
What are you doing this for?
Love.
Do there have to be answers?
No.
What is the point of being?
Everything.
What if you are already whole?
Okay.
All right.
Right now.
Please.
We move through our days
anyway
because
and now.
In an ocean of not knowing
there are undercurrents
of love and joy to
fuel your-my river of
being and becoming.
We're here.
Right now.

Mothers and Daughters

I woke thinking about mothers and daughters. I realize that I am both Persephone and Demeter in one. I am the daughter of my mother, the mother of my
daughter, and I am not quite what either of them wants me to be.

My daughter has an insatiable need for my companionship, my attention, my
exclusive focus, my time. I never feel like enough for her, I often feel like I am
letting her down in some way, never able to be all that she needs, never able to
give her everything she wants from me (which, perhaps, is everything). She is my
precious rainbow girl, my longed-for daughter, the baby who I almost gave up
on meeting. She is my only girl, the child that accompanied me through an Underworld journey of pregnancy loss, grief, and despair, the girl-child who healed
my heart when I thought it was broken forever. She was my happiest baby,
delight always radiating through her, my cherished reward after a year of agony.
We were inseparable. I felt like I mothered her *right,* the first baby to whom I
felt able to completely devote myself, to not feel like I needed a break from or
to escape from to restore some semblance of myself. We were a team: *the girls.*
Then, another brother arrived. My first unexpected pregnancy, one final boy to
round out our family into four children, three sons and one daughter. I feel like
my daughter has not ever forgiven me for this intrusion of the final brother into
our bond, the distance that was created by another body in my arms, another
love in my heart, another's need of me that trumped her own. He became my
baby and she became a big sister and she has not released the hurt of this betrayal
of my devotion to her.

All my kids need me. They all need my love and my time and my attention
and my validation. I am splintered into scraps, always trying and often failing, to
be enough for all of them, while also nurturing my business, paying attention to
our customers, meeting my obligations and responsibilities to my projects and
to other people. I told a friend recently that every morning when I wake up there
are five people in my immediate environment who I have a relationship with, to
whose relationship needs I must tend and nurture in some way. From the beginning of each day, that doesn't leave many other spaces in my relationship "energy
pool" to tend or to nourish or to nurture. I'm used up before I even begin.

My own mother is not disappointed in me—in who I *am* at least—but she,
too, lets me know in subtle and not so subtle ways that I don't spend enough
time with her, that maybe I work too much or am too devoted to our business.

This chronic time deficit I feel in my life as a whole, spills over to her as well, leaving her wishing for some of my time.

I recognize that I am at a low point in my hormonal cycle, approaching my moon time. This is when I feel the weariest, the most depleted, the most not-enough, and, often, I center this sensation on my parenting, identifying all the ways in which I have failed and disappointed and not given enough. I often decide at this point in the month that we're not doing enough schoolwork, that our parenting skills are deficient, that I should be spending even *more* time playing and entertaining...and then berating myself because I just *don't want to.*

It helps to recognize the hormonal connection and to recognize the pattern. I think back to my daughter's moment of birth and my cry of exultation to behold her in my blood-streaked hands: *you're okay, you're okay! There's nothing wrong with me!* Maybe I *am* still actually okay and there is nothing wrong with me.

> *And so the sun rises*
> *on a bright new day*
> *breathe in*
> *breathe out*
> *everything is okay...*

The Seventh Task

Our older sons are invited to a friend's house for an overnight and my mom invites the two younger children to spend the night at her house, leaving Mark and me free for an unexpected date night. This is a gift I hadn't realized we desperately needed.

The day is bright, sunny, and warm. The sky is clear blue and majestic. We decide to go for a ramble at the river land and explore through the woods, looking for deer antlers. We don't find any antlers, but we do spy the deer and also startle some wild turkeys who fly over the flooded creek bank looking encouragingly fat, shiny, and healthy. We follow a chickadee who leads us to a lone pine tree on the hillside, the only one we can see anywhere, tall and straight. A vulture circles overhead. Since we feel like we are friends now, we wave at it and call, *Hello, friend!* as it drifts in gentle circles on the air, never flapping its wings even once.

How might we float on the rhythms of this life as well? we muse.

We make our way out of the woods and back down the hillside and sit by the confluence of creek and river as sunset draws near. The vulture is circling over the field nearby now and then we see a bald eagle as well, following the river at first and then circling back through the field and over the tree. We startle a wood duck and then see two kingfishers. A small, charming purple finch interrupts our financial records overview and business-goal setting meeting that we've been hungering to find the time for. He settles on the ground near us, his little puff of a hairdo making us smile. He is businesslike and intent as he plucks leaves and debris off the ground, throwing things over his shoulder with a delightfully sassy attitude.

I am relieved to discover that life feels infinitely more simple and clear with some time by the river to think and be. The awareness creeps in that *maybe I am not actually having a breakdown, I just needed a break.* Sometimes when things feel difficult it is because they are. It is hard to run a successful business, to take care of myself, to tend to a marriage, to be a friend to others, to have employees in my house three days a week, and to take care of and homeschool four children. That is hard. The fact that it feels hard is because it *is, not* because there is something *inherently wrong* with me. I don't actually need to change my whole personality and, truly, I don't actually need to rearrange my whole life, I just need to take some time to look at the parts that feel painful and see what I might tweak or alter to allow ease in.

> *The seventh task*
> *is to take*
> *a break.*

Journeys

The sky is just beginning to show a stripe of red and a slender waning crescent moon hangs low above the horizon, bordered with shadowy clouds. The woods are quiet and I stand on the stones and cast a bubble of protection around the car, visualizing each person's face in turn and asking that we are protected, guarded, and surrounded with love as we travel, and are brought back home safely once more. I kneel and place my hands on the stones, drawing it up and sending it out. I do this every time we travel, rooting myself in the rhythms and safety of place and letting it carry me.

I feel like I need something more, like maybe this isn't enough. I let my shoulders drop and my hands fall open. The wind rises and stirs.

Persephone, please walk with me.

And then, two barred owls call from the trees, their voices rising together three times and then stopping.

Once again, I feel heard, received, witnessed.

I go back inside and drink some pomegranate juice with my yogurt for breakfast.

I step out on the deck one more time, as the sky lightens and the air becomes full of birdsong. I hear the phoebe and the twittering of many other birds. As we drive away, the fields are frosted white and mist rises over the river like smoke. Three deer cross in front of us, heading into the pine trees.

I must be clear that I do not think any of these animals are here *for me,* but I am humbled to witness them and to weave together my own meaning from their presence, to listen, to see, to hear, to be embedded *with them* in this magic, real world. The connections I find in these creatures of the sky to my questions, to my seeking, to the threads of the Goddess that weave through my days, feel mystical to me, while also being visceral, whole, resiliently present, and here. These animals are *with* me. They remind me to be present, here, alert, seeing, breathing, and feeling. They anchor me in magic, in the Goddess, in the purpose for being alive. They remind me that we are woven *together* in this tapestry of being, flying, and growing. We are all encircled.

I recall a quote from Phil Cousineau from his book *The Art of Pilgrimage: The Seeker's Guide to Making Travel Sacred:*

The time has come to set out for sacred ground that will stir our sense of wonder. It is down the path to the deeply real where time stops and we are seized by the mysteries. This is the journey that we cannot not take.

APRIL

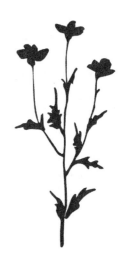

The Pendulum

We have made it to our first destination, the Smoky Mountains of Tennessee. I choose my Womanrunes card of the day and receive the Pendulum, the rune of patterns. Ah, yes! My pattern is making things difficult and denying ease.

My mind starts clicking though to all the things I need to take care of, that need me to pay attention to them, that "no one else" will handle unless I do. I make the grocery list and meal plan and then come inside feeling tight and disgruntled that everyone else is just hanging around in vacation mode waiting for me to push and remind and bug. I think about how tired I am of being the family "driver"—the motivator, the requester, the nagger, the pusher. I reflect on how I'm just carrying the same pattern from home, straight into vacation. The need to "get things done," the responsibility for making sure everyone is taken care of, the fulfillment of responsibilities before pleasure. I actually spend *less* time outside enjoying myself today while on vacation than I usually do while at home!

I sit on my yoga mat, watching the clouds over the mountains and suddenly realize that I could just *let it be easy.* I could just watch the clouds on the mountains today, that's it. If no one else wants to go anywhere, do anything, or get anything ready, why should I pester them to get moving?

I don't mean to confuse "ease" with abandonment or irresponsibility, but I continue to think,

*What if I could let it be easy, choose ease, in the moment? Not expecting it always, but recognizing it when it **is** an option and **allowing** it.*

This feels radical, again, like a departure from my habitual mode of engaging with life. *Isn't hard work necessary? Needed? Satisfying? If you just let things be easy, isn't that lazy, aren't you missing opportunities, or not fulfilling your potential? Taking the easy way out is a cop-out, isn't it? Isn't "easy" an excuse to stay small?* I still don't know. I think it *can* be those things, but I also know that I would like a feeling of *ease* within more often.

What if I just watched the clouds roll in?

I don't just watch the clouds roll in, though. I rally the crew and we depart on a series of errands that felt like they would be simple enough and yet manage to take the entire day, slurping it away in a morass of over-stimulating attractions. It is a constant clamor of light, sound, flash, consumption, and need in the town before the entrance to the Smoky Mountains National Park. There is so much to look at, so much trying to catch your eye and grab your dollar, that I feel as if we stumble around in a daze.

I keep my eyes out for birds. I know the birds will anchor me within myself even though they fly without anchor. We see three ducks flying low as we stagger through a giant parking lot to an overlit, overpriced shopping center. I don't even remember to say my "Persephone, please walk with me" prayer, I'm too dazed and visually overwhelmed, energetically taxed. It is the first day of my moon time and I feel like drawing inward. My patience feels thin and I am strained from travel and cognitively at a low ebb. I have an excruciating headache that builds to a throbbing stab. I scrabble an old Advil out of my purse, and it does help with the pain, but I still feel dull and unfocused.

We finally drive back to our little apartment with its beautiful mountain-view balcony on the top floor. *Why did we leave? Why did we do this to ourselves?* We are not sure. It is like we got sucked down into the quicksand of the lights and signs and promises. We also didn't want to have to go back out into the strip again, we wanted to get it over with in one fell swoop, instead of revisiting the experience on any of our other days. No one is happy. We are all snippy and disappointed with one another and our experiences and choices.

Even though we need to cook dinner, Mark and I decide to head out for a walk before sunset. I'm so grateful we are staying somewhere with a view, somewhere reasonably quiet, somewhere with a balcony, many tall trees, and birds. We admire the redbud blossoms and find a crabapple tree and smell its flowers. The cold air burns my lungs as we walk up a steep paved hill. I feel my sense of soul coming back to me. I'm not sure why I become so diffuse, so unseated, so unmoored, when in highly populated areas, but I do. I know I should have taken better care of my own energy today, should have watched those clouds, listened to the wisdom about old patterns, let it be easy.

Reflection

The morning dawns bright and beautiful. I take my green tea to the solace of the balcony and settle down with my journals and Womanrunes cards. I draw Reflection, rune of surrender and letting go.

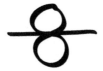

This is what I crave. Time to reflect. Time to be still and think and be and write and learn. Time to let go of my old patterns and behaviors and habits of mind. I look up just in time to see a crow sweep across the valley. It is quiet, but some of its unseen friends are cawing in welcome.

Persephone, please walk with me.

I write for a few minutes and then look up to see a vulture rising and falling above the distant Smokies. As I watch, enchanted by the grace and ease of its coasting path, two and then briefly, three, more vultures join the dance. They glide and coast, coming in and out of view in the blue-gray sky and clouds above the mountains. It is like a dance, a graceful, beautiful, peaceful, magical dance. Again, I feel like I could stay here all day, just watching this one patch of mountains and what lives within my view.

But I don't stay all day.

We decide to go on a hike to Laurel Falls. Traffic is horrendous. I do see a crow, carrying something in its beak. Perhaps I should have taken it as a sign to go back! There is so much traffic, there is nowhere to park and we decide to drive on.

We eventually discover a small hiking trail off the beaten path with empty parking places. We park and set off on what becomes a four-mile hike. We only see three other families the entire time (on our way back) and we finally feel like we are doing something right. The sun is shining brightly, the sky is clear, the mountains and trees are beautiful. The kids are a little whiny, but it is okay, we are hiking in the Smokies, just like we planned!

We walk on a ridge of reality
between civilization
and wildness
in a land of
shadowed hollows
and mountain laurel
where cathedraled pines
form the only monuments
and great slabs of mountain
bones
stand sentinel over tiny cities
woven of root
and time.
We lose count of the crows
that guide the way to the
next secret
and the names of babies
etched in crumbling stone
tell of forgotten sorrows
and timeworn worries
in a valley of unknown stories.
I plunge my arms
into newborn waters
older than the hills
and let the current wash away
my expectations

It is good to be alive and breathing
in this woods-rapt
point of eternity and change.

Today We Soften

Today, we soften.

We finally realize that this area of the country, at the time we have chosen, is just too crowded for us to enjoy. We let go of our plans to hike a small part of the Appalachian Trail in the park. We let go of the waterfall. We even let go of the easy downtown walking trail, after we attempt to drive to it and are stuck in bumper-to-bumper traffic.

We go swimming in the saltwater pool at the resort and enjoy sitting in the saltwater hot tub looking out at the mountains. We spot a wild turkey crossing the parking lot, a hawk in a distant pine, three vultures circling high in the sky, and a crow, always a crow, flying over the trees.

As I watch the crows from the hot tub, I realize that it is my worry that I *should* be doing something different, should be going to the right places, doing the right things, seeing the right sights, that is hampering this trip more than anything else. Once I unclench my fists, I realize that truly, I just want to sit on the balcony and look at the mountains and that is all I've wanted to do, really, since we got here—and, yet, as is too often my default pattern at home too, I deny myself the thing I truly want, either putting it off until later or when the work is all done or, worse yet, never doing it at all because I run out of time for what I actually want to do, after taking care of everything else that needs me.

Even today, I don't actually sit on the balcony until it is dusk and dinner is later than it should be. The balcony feels too simple, like not enough, like we didn't drive all this way and spend this money just to sit on a balcony and look at the mountains. And so, I see, I've spent hardly any time doing the thing I genuinely most want to do in favor of attempting to do things that I think I ought to want to do, but that no one in my family is enjoying.

I light a candle and sit on the balcony in the deepening night, watching the clouds over the mountains fade to a darkness that eventually absorbs the mountains into the clouds.

I watched three vultures dance
over the Smoky Mountains
rising and falling,
dipping and weaving
in languid, leisurely,
lovely circles
buoyed by their own knowing
that they may glide
on the support
that surrounds them
as they appear and disappear
in turns into cool
gray-blue clouds.
We could learn a lot
from vultures:
Waste nothing.
Coast when you can.
Trust the support
beneath you.
Soar as high as possible.
Play with the wind.

Thank You

Tanner crawls into bed with us right before I'm ready to get up. I curl my fingers around his skinny little arm and feel a clench in my heart at his still-smallness. This is the tail-end of babyness in my life, the last year of being needed in that wholehearted, body-based, intensive mothering way. I've spent fifteen years doing this so far, in some ways I feel utterly spent and burned out, in others I feel like it is over before it began. Just when I've finally, sort of, figured out what I'm doing and how to live with being needed this way, it is done.

I go out onto the balcony with my green tea and watch the mist curling around the mountains, it looks like it is climbing the trees, dipping and swirling like a river. I hear crows from multiple directions, but can't spot them.

While in the saltwater hot tub last night, I was thinking about how I must have a moment of enchantment in every day, how I must feel magic to feel alive. Is this spoiled or self-centered? *Is it unrealistic to expect magic every day?* I don't actually think it is. The world would likely be a better place if each person allowed their soul to be fueled by the magic of living. I don't need much to feel the magic, but I do need to feel it. And despite the challenges and disappointments of our experiences here so far, there has been magic in every one of our days. Thank Goddess I know to look for the birds.

After the whirlwind of packing for the next destination, the raised voices, the chaos, the last-minute trips to the bathroom, I decide to step out on the balcony one last time.

Despite everything, thank you for being here, I say.

I look to my right and there is a lone crow sitting in the bare limbs of a dead pine tree, against the backdrop of mystical cloud cover blanketing the mountains.

Thank you. Thank you.

> *What if this was the year*
> *you actually let yourself*
> *have what you want?*
> *Not just occasional treats,*
> *or little gifts*
> *or one walk in the woods.*
> *What if you leaned fully into desire*
> *and met it all the way?*
> *What if you paid attention to the whispers,*
> *to the hum of longing,*
> *to the way your bones know what you need?*
> *What if you trusted yourself enough to really*
> *live your life,*
> *to savor your deepest yeses*
> *and your most honorable nos,*
> *embodying your joy,*
> *feeling the magic that is alive*
> *in you every day,*
> *asking to be heard.*
> *What if you let yourself dream*
> *right now*

of what your life could look like,
of what you could hold,
of what it might feel like to shed
the bonds of have to, must do,
force and fatigue?
What if you already know exactly what you need?
What if you trust it?
What if you say yes
to yourself?

New Moon on Myrtle Beach

Our drive to South Carolina is relatively easy, first driving through impressive mountains bordered by broad rivers in North Carolina and then the landscape flattens as we cross South Carolina to the sea.

The next morning I wake to birds singing and the sound of the waves. The atmosphere is peaceful here and I feel at home on the shore. We set off at sunrise for a walk along the shore and end up walking for five miles. Myrtle Beach is more crowded with high-rise buildings and more populous than we are used to at Dauphin Island in Alabama, where we go each year. But there is something about the ocean that creates spaciousness and peace, no matter what.

I stand in the waves and realize that when you are facing the ocean, filled with her sound, it doesn't really matter how many other people are around, there is still a sensation of solitude. I watch the clouds. I watch the seagulls. I listen to the waves. I feel the cool water sweeping over my ankles and drawing the sand from beneath my feet over and over again, necessitating that I keep adjusting my feet, on these shifting sands of life and time.

I watch a quartet of college student-age girls taking photographs on the beach. I remember being that age, both self-conscious and unconscious of parts of myself and my relationships with others. They pose and re-pose and pose again, always running around to squint at the tiny screen after each shot.

I notice how these girls are not actually *present*. They are going through the motions—the act, the pose—of being here, but they aren't really here, and they aren't really doing anything. They are setting up a scene, staging an experience, pretending to have fun for the camera. I think about times in which I have done the same—getting the picture versus having the experience. I become aware of myself as the observer, noticing my own judgments and noticing that if I'm focused on evaluating the hereness of others, I'm not really *here* either! I watch the artfully arranged jut of the hip, the flip of the hair, the frequent adjustment of the bikini tops, the toned bodies, the carefully casual glances and "sexy" faces. I think about the male gaze—remembering how it can be both predatory to experience and powerful to command. I am almost forty now and I am becoming more aware of how I have benefited from the privileges of youth, relative attractiveness, and relative thinness throughout my own life. How I am sometimes conscious, but more often unconscious, of how a big smile full of straight teeth, can open doors, smooth conflicts, and invite trust.

My daughter runs over to me and asks me to play in the waves with her. She is getting taller and only has a few years left before she might become aware of what it means to experience the male gaze too—both the predation and the pleasure and power of it. Today, though, she is a Maiden on the Shore, fully present, fully herself, unselfconscious, and whole. She has not been told how to be or who she can be, she has not yet seen herself through the eyes of others and found herself wanting or lacking in some way. I feel fierce and protective of her. I wish for her this easy grace in her own skin always, without the messages of culture and society etching upon it their own wishes and needs, eroding her sense of self and courage, dictating her choices and the cock of her hip, the calculated flip of her hair and arch of her back.

While the Triple Goddess archetype is widely criticized as too narrow and confining for the breadth and depth of most women's lived realities, I can also recognize that my life is in fact divided into three distinct stages. Before menarche and after menarche are distinctly recognizable in my memory. When I first began Red Tent work and meditated on the Maiden in my own life, I was shocked to discover that there is a clear division in my body-mind between *before* menstruation and *after* menstruation, and that *after* feels like it involves less happiness and more confusion and angst and an altered relationship to my body and how much I trust her. I remember myself as carefree, happy, and at ease in myself prior to menstruation and also eagerly awaiting her arrival. Post-menstruation I recall the intensely painful cycles I experienced, the feeling as if I was "sick" when I had my period, and no longer feeling in blissful harmony with my body, no longer able to run with abandon and be fully free again. Giving birth in power and joy helped me reclaim my body trust and delight (and eased the symptoms of my cycles), but it took another ten years for me to recognize that my ongoing moon cycle might hold sacred wisdom and opportunities for insight and divine connection.

Giving birth and becoming a mother is also a distinct, transformative, and initiatory rite in my own life. As with menstruation, there is a definite distinction between *before motherhood* and *after motherhood.* And, in many ways, I am not the same person I was before going through this rite of transformation.

While I am not yet in the Crone stage I can sense that this will be similar, only it will likely represent the division between life as a mother with children at home and life as a mother with adult children, as well as an evolving conception of myself and my relationship to my own body and her capacities.

I watch four vultures wheeling in the gray clouds above the high rises on the beach.

What am I still shedding, releasing, and cleansing from my life?

There is still so much to let go.

It is new moon and I decide to make my collage goddess for March. Each month this year near the new moon, I make one with the themes, messages, and imagery of the preceding month. At the end of the year, I will then have a set of twelve wooden collage goddesses that visually depict the lessons and explorations of the year. The background for this month's, cut from a seed catalog, providentially has three strips of different kinds of flowers and a young girl's face at the bottom, perfect for my Maiden contemplations. I add some crows and a full moon, cut from an old We'Moon datebook. On the head of the goddess, I put a hawk, wheeling through blue skies over stalks of waving wheat. I combine some lines from one of my own poems into a slightly new form:

> *You come to a*
> *crossroads*
> *of being.*
> *There*
> *you discover*
> *your heart,*
> *conduit of*
> *the holy.*
> *Time to coax*
> *your truth*
> *out of hiding.*

At sunset, I take my new crystals down to the waves to cleanse them. This feels fitting for the new moon. I bend and dip each one gently in the water, the sand glowing a light pink as the sun sets behind the tall buildings.

May I let go.
May I release habits of mind and patterns of
thought that are no longer helpful.
May I shed what needs to be shed.
May I be cleansed and renewed.
May these stones support me in new beginnings
and in standing in my own power.

The first slender crescent of the new moon appears low in the sky, between the tall buildings. It always makes my breath catch when the moon (of any phase) "suddenly" appears in this way—like it has just winked into existence at that moment, or is specifically saying hello, answering a question, or responding to a prayer.

Look for the next new beginning
and welcome it.
Look for the next opportunity
to persist
and celebrate it.
Look for the tiniest moment
in which the sacred sings.
Look for the softest, smallest magic
you can find.
Look for the enchantment
humming invisibly
beneath the surface of each thing.
Let the tides shift and the pages turn
and look for your place
within the changes and ripples
of this uncertain and beautiful life.

Persephone's Song

I decide to go for a morning walk alone as Mark is unwell. It feels strange at first to be doing our favorite thing alone, but soon I settle into the rhythm. I think about how close Persephone felt in the woods at home and how the Goddess as I know her in general feels more distant at the beach, because there is another presence here—the broader and more universal Goddess perhaps, but not the same force as that which inhabits the green spaces and stony places.

Persephone, please walk with me.

I say it aloud and with more cadence than I have before and for the first time, I recognize that my little prayer rhymes. I start to sing it gently under my breath and before I know it, other lines roll obligingly in.

> *Through shadowed lands*
> *with outstretched hands.*
> *Across hills and vales*
> *in unknown tales.*
> *Through chambers*
> *of the Underworld*
> *through stories*
> *that are rarely told.*

I sing these sets of lines for a while as I listen to the gulls and the waves and watch the pelicans.

> *With patient heart*
> *and seeds of glee*
> *Persephone*
> *please walk with me.*

A few other lines come to mind. These feel insistent, demanding almost, they *need* to be incorporated into my song. I don't usually use phrases like, "My guides told me" or, "The Goddess asked me." But that is what this feels like. As if Persephone is asking for specific parts of the song. *Honeyed hair,* I hear over and over. Then, *plains of power.* I weave these into the song as I continue to sing and walk. At three points, I stop to finish a line, feeling it out in the context of the rest of the song, stopping and standing to feel if I've gotten it *right*.

I look down to discover a moon snail right at my feet.

I turn around to come back, I've already walked two miles, singing almost the entire time. I worry briefly that I will lose the song, facing the other direction without having written it down, but instead I receive another of those insistent lines:

Past shades of what will never be.

I even try to change it, but it wants, *she* wants, those exact words.

More imagery rushes in. I can see us now, setting out across misty trails, up hills, and into valleys, through groves and into smoky dens and forgotten caves, by rivers to the sea, and across plains of power and chambers of the Underworld. The visual imagery is so vivid that I again have the sensation I felt by the lake in town at home, like I've reached out, across, and through time, to touch this thread of Persephone's own experience. I think about how I have not perceived her as a "powerful" goddess, but rather, as in my song, a companion goddess. However, like each of us who journeys through this life, Persephone is powerful, and I sense that power, that steadfastness and determination, in my song as well.

Persephone
please walk with me
through shadowed lands
with outstretched hands.
Across hills and vales
in unknown tales.
Through dells
and dales
on misty trails.
Past sunny glades
and shady glens
straight up to
smoky, swirling dens.
Through foggy groves,
past quiet graves,

into the long
forgotten caves.
Through chambers of
the Underworld
through stories
that are rarely told.
Across plains of power
and pain-swept hours
by singing brooks
and mossy nooks.
Past shades of
what will never be
by rivers stretching
to the sea.
Through valleys
of timeworn care
with steady steps
and honeyed hair.
With silent prayers
on red-stained lips
and flowers
on your fingertips.
With patient heart
and seeds of glee,
Persephone
please walk with me.

The Eighth Task

The day is foggy and overcast, but I can hear the waves from the bed. Mark is still feeling terrible, but he walks with me for about half a mile. I continue for another four miles without him, I go back over my Persephone song, streamlining it down to the original series of lines that first came to me and that are easier to remember and sing in full than the extended version. I sing it over and over again as I walk.

I reach the beach marker labeled '33' and once again find a worn but whole moon snail shell waiting for me, right in the same spot. I'm surprised at how quickly we make these discoveries and how predictable these seemingly unpredictable patterns are. I see two crows again and I feel like there is something here waiting for me, maybe I *will* discover a big shell on this beach after all. I find several more whole, worn moon snails. They are small though and I always want large ones.

I end up going in the water up to my knees seeking an elusive something I feel is here. I catch myself as I wait for the story, for *the* moment.

I start the story multiple times, only to find nothing. I do find two small, shiny lettered olive shells rolling by beneath the waves, but that is it. I laugh at myself a bit and how I am always waiting for the story, always alert to the story in the moments. Sometimes there doesn't have to be a story, I think. *Why do I even expect a story?* I realize two things with this question:

1. I have a story worth telling (so do you!)

2. There is magic everywhere.

I have been honored and privileged enough to experience something magical in just about every day of the last two years (which is when I started keeping track of magical daily moments in my journal). I look for the magical moment, for the story of the things connecting and me witnessing it, because I have been fortunate enough to see and experience time and time again that it is *there. Why shouldn't I expect the story?*

I am writing myself back into being. I am writing my soul back into herself. I am looking for the story because I know it is there and because it is how I am rebuilding myself, word by word, step by step, shell by shell. Feminist theorist Mary Daly created the word "be-speaking," which she defines as:

Bringing about a psychic and/or material change by means of words, speaking into being. To be-speak an invocation, you must be fully present with what you are saying.[*]

---

[*] digitalcommons.lsu.edu/cgi/viewcontent.cgi?article=6863&context=gradschool_disstheses

A personal friend, Cynthia Cebuar, adds that:

Another way of saying it is to inhabit the words as they inhabit you—the "feeling it in your bones" kind of experience. Let the words arise out of the lips of the Goddess who resides within you and speak to Her who also resides without.

I think about how I am keeping this story, this journey, close to my heart instead of rushing to share. I'm so used to reporting everything, of packaging it into a social media post, but this feels tender and vulnerable. Rebuilding the soul is a private process, largely an internal one, while at the same time with a significant external component, since it involves paying deep attention and making connections between what is happening on the inside and what is happening on the outside, around you.

I recognize that I do feel confused about the next step.

What am I supposed to do now in this journey of rebuilding my soul?

How will I know what to do next?

What do I even want? What do I actually need? What am I expecting?

Am I actually accomplishing anything or doing any work in this process or am I still figuring out what, if anything, this process is?

I start speaking aloud, some poem-thoughts about what I even mean by rebuilding the soul. This work, perhaps, *can* be distilled into some key lessons, key points, and I *am* doing this work.

I walk under the pier, speaking the lines of my newly born poem quietly out loud to myself, and feel a warm splat on my shoulder. The poem flies out of my mind as I look over my shoulder to discover a fresh, hot deposit of bird poop on my shoulder, running down my new t-shirt and onto the top of my arm. This is the first time I have ever been pooped on by a bird, and, ironically, just as I was waxing eloquent about enchantment and soul-rebuilding. I discover I've completely forgotten my new poem, it has been eclipsed by this warm, spreading stain. I go back to find my family to show them the poop, laughing and jolted so firmly back into the present that I'm actually grateful to this bird and this poop.

> *The eighth task*
> *is to remember*
> *to laugh.*

Recipe for Rebuilding a Soul

When I get back to the resort I am trying to remember my earlier "wisdom," pre-bird poop. I can't get it back, the insight has fled. But, I start to get something else, a recipe for soul rebuilding. I keep getting new pieces of it, climbing out of the hot tub repeatedly to add new lines.

Recipe for Rebuilding a Soul:

1 weary heart
2 open arms
1 large flat rock
As many tall pine trees
as you can find
1 empty book
Many pens
Lots of water
2 scoops of sunlight
An infinity of starshine.

Mix together patiently and wait in the shadows. Let rise in the sun. Let rise with the moon. Check for delight. If still soggy and deflated, expose on a hillside or soak in the ocean. Sprinkle with laughter.

Submerge beneath a stream of inspiration.
Drizzle with dreams and a generous helping of time.
Steep with incredible slowness.
Dust with flowers and (k)nee(a)d well.
Let become exquisitely tender and soft.

When fully risen, warmed throughout, and glowing with strength and satisfaction, enjoy with a tall glass of moonlight, a side of magic, and a handful of enchantment.

Create regularly for best results.

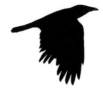

After I add the final lines, I lean back in the hot tub and see that there are two crows flying over my head.

Messages

I have a strong sensation that the crows are carrying messages for me, but that perhaps I'm not quite listening well enough, or that I'm somehow overlooking the point.

I'm not sure what to do with the sensation that I'm supposed to be learning or doing something specific, like something is *palpably* waiting for me to figure it out, to discover it. I can sense a next step close by. *Or, is it very possible that I am doing it right now, feeling my way, uncovering the path bit by bit, discerning my tasks, applying my lessons, listening, and listening again?*

I am struck by an insight from Jack Kornfield that I recently discovered via Jennifer Louden, *"a state of mind is always temporary."* There is nothing to achieve permanently. I will never be able to completely "fix" myself and always do it right all the time. What I really want to do, after I "get it," is carry it with me and *apply* it, recognizing enoughness and honoring it, instead of overriding it.

> *Keep returning to your body.*
> *Keep returning to your breath.*
> *Keep returning to your heart.*
>
> *What do you actually want?*
> *What do you actually hear?*
>
> *Listen. Do. Feel. Be.*

I find, as I write this book, that I am approaching each day with a sense of curiosity and anticipation that I *get* to witness, experience, encounter, explore, and describe *what happens next*. Every day I wait to find out, every day I look for (and experience) the next part of my own story.

Before bed, I read some of *The Mist-Filled Path* by Frank MacEowen and think about pilgrimages and Heroine's Journeys of descent, initiation, and renewal. The author writes about the process of initiation, as unfolding moments of discovery, exploration, and longing, which is exactly what I feel like is happening to me right now. He explains:

Nearly all initiations, if they are truly centered in the life of the soul, are about stepping into right relationship with the spirit of longing. Initiation is the process of defining and refining one's role in the life of our longing, determining how we can be conduits for its influence in our lives and world. Regardless of the number of visions, tutelages, advance degrees, or sacred objects that may have entered our lives, if we forget to listen to the voice of longing, we will get nowhere.

It occurs to me that I could do some research on the Heroine's Journey, on personal quests, on myths of descent and renewal. At the same time, I realize that I am not interested in researching paths or studying traditions, developing theories, or forming plans or programs, or even drawing conclusions or making pronouncements. I just want to watch the rainbows dance in the water and to feel my bones against the grass. These tasks I have discerned as I move through these organic, initiatory processes of discovery, *am I truly living into and through them?*

> *Expect to be enchanted.*
> *Show up and pay attention.*
> *Hold your wonder with tender fingers.*
> *Be patient.*
> *Watch for signs.*
> *Take time.*
> *Make time.*
> *Feel it all.*
> *Be more patient.*
> *Wait.*

Say yes to breathing easy
and to wandering.
Bleed if you need to.
Curl up.
Spread out.
Be still.
Move.
Wait some more.
Hope with your arms
wide open.
Expect magic to find you
and when she does
say yes,
I will,
and thank you.

Pink

I find myself thinking about a dream I had many years ago, but that remains with me as one of the most significant cosmological events of my life.

*I am walking down to the woods behind my house when I discover that in the sky above the priestess rocks, where I stand each morning, there is a gigantic, beautiful, pulsating, pink, jeweled rose-like flower. I am awe-struck. It is the most beautiful thing I have ever seen. I become aware that a golden cord stretches from the center of the flower to the top of my head, and that all people are connected to the same flower by these golden cords. Then, in that uniquely expansive character of dreams, I somehow travel through the center of the flower. On the other side is an immense snake of unimaginable proportion, spiraling around the "cosmic egg." As I look at it, I become aware that the snake is actually the whole of the universe and that along its body, in the scales, one could perceive not only each galaxy, but also a point for **all times and places that ever were or will be.***

It is hard to describe in writing, but I still deeply remember my feelings of awe and comprehension and an expansive awareness of reality. It was a gorgeous, trippy, and meaningful dream. I tried to draw something about it, but was unable to do so. Instead, I was left with a feeling of majesty, magnitude, and incredible connection, that I can still recall with vivid intensity, even though many years have since passed.

I have let go of some control this month in my local women's circle, which I have priestessed with such love, care, and planning over the last ten years. I asked for volunteers to plan our April Pink Moon Pink Tent Circle[*] and several women have enthusiastically and spiritedly risen to the task and are making the plans largely without my input. I am noticing other people being capable, shining, and rising to the occasion, and it feels good to step back and allow this unfolding, rather than feeling completely responsible for it. I wonder how often my own sensation of responsibility as well as my own capability has interfered with or overshadowed what others might have to contribute.

> *When it is safe*
> *to say enough*
> *I am satisfied*
> *instead of fried,*
> *heart-centered*
> *instead of heart-sore,*
> *content instead of coerced,*
> *at ease instead of accelerated.*
> *I am undoing my knots.*

Tender Scars

Today we walk for about three miles, finding a few small shells and talking. Our thoughts turn to freedom and whether or not any of our choices can be truly "free," or are they always constrained, shaped, by the needs of others. It is sobering to consider the illusion of choice coupled with the reality of how often those choices are shaped by our environment, access, relationships, and even physical

---

[*] A variation on a Red Tent circle for girls and their mothers.

capacities. Mark mentions feeling as if he doesn't have a passion area of his own, that he would like to develop something that is for himself. He reflects that what we are doing with our business is mostly in service to my vision, my passion, and he doesn't really have something that belongs to him. I say that if I am the fuel of our business, if I am the passion that drives us and moves us and motivates us, what am I supposed to do now that my fire is fading, that my drive is quieting, that I'm burning out on being the fuel? As he always does when I bring this up, he doesn't answer, but lets my questions slide away into the waves.

I try to talk about it again in the car on the way back to the resort — *where do we go, or what do we choose if I feel like my fire is being extinguished?* Again, the words hang heavy in the air between us and his attention slides away from me, leaving my questions weighty and unwelcome. I feel unexpected tears prickling behind my eyes and we continue in silence, the words still there, until they finally fade into silence and he starts a different conversation.

Back at the room, I tell him that I feel like he avoids engaging when I talk about feeling burned out, but that if, as a business, we rely on my steam and energy, it is something we *have* to be willing to address or we will extinguish me, put out the fire of our biggest asset. He finally says that when he hears me say things like this, he feels accused of not doing enough for our business, of not working hard enough, when really, he puts everything he has into it. While I still feel the unresolved questions, I am glad to have an opportunity to explain that my feelings have nothing to do with what he is doing, but with my own capacities and whether or not my current choices, workload, and means of engagement are sustainable (they aren't!).

I am making progress here, but I still have quite a way to go, as I have knots to untie from forty years of conditioning and habit-forming. It feels, sometimes, that this is how I have done everything of worth in my life — pushed it — even when I'm weary and heart-sore, I keep pushing. The aspect that is difficult to reconcile is that I also know that this pushing has sometimes produced works of great beauty and joy: our four children, multiple books, and a business that sustains our whole family and three employees as well.

I think briefly of the births of my children, and remember that three of them slipped effortlessly from my body with no active pushing or strain, once I set my mind aside and let my body do the work. Each one also left a scar upon my tenderest, most private flesh, forever changing my experience of my body and her capacity to function.

Belonging

As I walk the shore this afternoon, I think about the land, I think about the ir-resistible call of the ocean to me and how much I love it at the beach. I am won-dering if our time of living in the woods is actually ready to draw to a close, even though the woods have shaped my life and spirituality so profoundly (I feel like I've betrayed a trust even by typing this). *Is there something in me that compels me to the sea? Am I meant to be near the water?* I think about how entwined my life is with the land I live on — the land I was born and raised on, the land on which seven generations of my family have breathed and walked and bled and cried. The land, the woods of Missouri, are in my bones and blood. They are my homeland, my birthplace, my habitat, my bloodland. But the ocean... There is something in these waves.

I start to think about ancestry and colonization and how my further-distant people did *not "come from" these shores, but from other lands and other seas. Were they invaders and conquerors? Did they slash and burn their way across the land, or did they tend to sacred groves with tender fingers? Did they love the soil they stood on? Did they nourish life and health and peace?*

I think of my own gentle father and my creative mother, and then my moth-er's ambitious, powerful father and her talented, creative, adventurous mother. I think of my father's hard-working, tenacious father and his quiet, funny mother. I think of my father's ancestors, hailing from Scotland and Ireland and England. *What brought my people to what became my homeland, the place of my roots, my birth, my heart?* I do not know. And there is certainly no remnant of Scottish or Irish tradition remaining in the conscious awareness of my family. My DNA is thoroughly European and yet here I stand, on North American shores, feeling bound here thoroughly by my blood and bones.

I wonder about these other lands from which my actual genes derive — *does it have anything to do with the call of the sea and the joy of green moss on stony hillsides?* I extend my awareness to these nameless ones, on the lands they loved and died on, the weaving of their lives through time and into mine.

Persephone as Lover

Before we depart this morning, I offer a small handful of rose petals, pineapple sage, and lavender to the land we are leaving. I recognize a feeling of disconnection from my magic today with another long drive to our next destination, so I remember my own advice and look for the birds.

Today, I don't feel like I'm paying enough attention, like I'm missing something. I'm not as present or alert as I could be. I see robins, a hawk, vultures, turning in the sky over quickly-forgotten streets in similar cities. I feel curious about my next steps, I wonder about the next element, the next goddess, and when I will receive my next mission. *Which element will be next?* I feel like it will be Water, but in the wheel of the year and it should really be Fire. I will wait to find out.

Perhaps one of the things I need to learn to do is wait. Wait and see. Wait and learn. Wait and be.

I feel as if I'm not only undoing, or attempting to undo, my own knots, I'm trying to reprogram or re-pattern my habitual ways of thinking or experiencing or responding. And, what I recognize as I write is that I need to apply the tasks and messages I've already been given, I need to live into and through them, I need to remember, even in stressful moments, that which I've committed to, that which I have uncovered and discovered, that which has already been revealed to me. Perhaps I will actually spend *all year* working with Air, the birds are definitely not finished with me yet. When we arrive at our next stop in the Blue Ridge Mountains of North Carolina, I step out onto the balcony and immediately see a crow flying away to the left. I hear another crow to the right and then see one directly in front of me. Three crows. I am here.

Later, as I rise to meet my husband's body after a long "dry spell," I think of Persephone as a lover, as a woman freely choosing her love and offering her body, dripping with honey and flowering beneath strong, wandering hands. She is most often identified as a maiden goddess, a daughter goddess, and then an Underworld Queen, but hidden beneath the more classic stories, we may find a love story between a dark god and a maiden goddess. When I teach *Cakes for the Queen of Heaven,* my friends and I replay the feminist vision of Persephone's journey, how she spots the dark man watching her in the flowers, how she falls in love with him and visits him secretly in a leafy bower, how she plans to leave the binding pull of mother-daughter love and follower her lover. Once in the

Underworld, she takes in the pomegranate seeds—the seeds of Hades—and flourishes with love and passion into someone surer of herself, capable and potent, an Underworld Queen. And she navigates between the worlds *because* of love.

There are words that come to me in this stolen hour with Mark as my lover instead of my teammate or co-planner, but they fade quickly, feeling like they were breathed to me across time—words of love and shadows and choice and rosy bowers and sticky thighs and consuming passion.

Ancient Tiny Cities

At Linville Falls we hike to three overlooks. As we emerge from the trail, a yellow butterfly floats lightly in the air above a mossy tree stump—*be light,* she seems to remind me. We find tiny perfectly curled fiddlehead ferns lining one mossy segment of the path and as I stoop to photograph them, I hear:

> *Where fiddleheads*
> *are gently furled*
> *you know there's magic*
> *in the world.*

And I do know. There are purple violets and yellow dandelions blooming all along the trails, as well as another smaller yellow flower I don't recognize. There are ancient tiny cities woven of root and time here too. Many fallen trees are carpeted with such glorious expanses of moss. Each one looks like a potential doorway to another world. I want to stop and photograph every one.

A partially fallen tree forms a threshold over the trail, its intricate root structure joining with the roots of another tree still holding it in place, alive, though it is nearly horizontal above the trail. Passing through this threshold feels like entering into something, I'm not sure what, but I do know a liminal doorway when I see one.

> *In curve of root*
> *and arc of stone*

there is a place
for dreams
to roam.

The Falls are huge and roaring, pounding through an astonishing water-hewn gorge of giant boulders. There are pigeons on the edge of the gorge and a pair of mourning doves flies out of the woods in front of us. I am filled with glee and excitement to be out and exploring. I feel like this walk heals the disappointment we experienced with our thwarted attempts to see the waterfalls in the Smokies. *This is what I imagined doing here,* I tell Mark with delight, standing in the sensation of being at the edge of water meeting air, meeting earth, over rocks once forged by fire.

Watch how it all weaves together and be astonished, I write in my journal as we continue to drive.

We get to our destination, a gemstone mining location called Emerald Village. We sit on the bench by the gem sluice, the six of us in a row, and sort through our bucket of gem rough.

When we were here before, I was early in my second trimester of my pregnancy with Alaina, and full of fear about losing another baby. I remember sitting here nine years ago feeling an insistent twinge of pain right above my pubic bone and realizing I had a bladder infection. The only other bladder infection of my entire life was at this exact same point in pregnancy with a baby who died. I ended up calling my rarely-seen family doctor's office in Missouri and they called a prescription for antibiotics in to a nearby Wal-Mart in North Carolina. I remember hurrying to pick up the antibiotics feeling a very real sensation that I was *saving my baby.*

It feels good to be here again, with that baby now a tall, funny, Pokémon-playing girl with wavy hair, deep blue eyes, and braces on her top teeth. *Did I save her that day as I followed my instincts and that twinge in my belly?* I don't know for sure, but I do remember how she saved me from my sorrow, my despair, and my eroded sense of body trust following the death of her tiny, older brother, Noah, and then the miniature lost embryo that came after him only three months later.

We stop by the same Wal-Mart to pick out a box of ice cream treats for the kids. As we walk through the store, I realize that I am feeling a stab of pain repeatedly, low in my belly, right above my pubic bone. Body memories are incredibly powerful.

We walk to the former mine on the property, a deep, round cave in the center of a mountain. Right as we approach, I notice there is a shaft of illuminated mist coming from one cavern within and pointing into another cavern directly across from it. It reminds me viscerally of an ancient temple, constructed in an astrologically perfect way to deliver a message, to teach a lesson, or to facilitate a spiritual experience. We turn away to set up a family photo and then I decide I'd like to take a goddess picture with the shaft of light. I had assumed it must be a regular geological feature here, but when I turn back with my goddess in my hand, it is gone as if it had never been there.

We get one free gem cut with our gem bucket at the mine and I choose an interesting looking three-layered stone that looks like Tiger's Eye, but is blue and white. They tell me it is called Hawk's Eye. In the shop on site, I buy a small carved stone bead shaped like a crow.

Later, at our small villa, we go out on the balcony to lay out our stones. As soon as I step out the door, a crow flies directly across the horizon in front of me.

Be Too Awake

We wake to rain and a dark building with no electricity and no cell phone access. I find myself thinking about social media and how fragmenting and distracting it can be. Now, without access to my morning scroll and "catch up" I stare out the glass door in the bedroom at the cloudy trees, still almost bare in this part of the country, instead of glowing with flowers and the blush of green we saw when we were further south.

Staring at raindrops and swaying gray branches and listening to the wind, induces a sort of calm reverie that isn't possible when I reach for a phone in all my down moments, even if what I'm using it for is answering customer messages, communicating with our community via social media, or tending to another of the many "real" and valuable tasks I do through the medium.

Writing in a continuous narrative instead of immediately posting about it, is guarding something precious to me, changing the texture of how I relate to the world, but also to the form and shape of my own life. I am enjoying the release from feeling compelled to produce for consumption. I am enjoying holding something close, working on something from within, instead of being consumed.

I step briefly onto the rainy deck, the mist is thick, and the wind swirls my hair up and around my face. I find it constantly reinforced for me that the elements are here to greet us, the magic is here to greet us, if we're willing to step into it and to be aware, attentive, and engaged. There is so much that wants to be whispered on the wind.

We leave this resort for the final destination of our trip and three crows graze the small greenway by the side of the road as we hit the highway again. I am ready to go home. I have enjoyed our trip and the many experiences we have shared, but I feel a longing in my heart for the grounded connection of my own space, the land to which I belong, the land I know and the land that knows me. I am rooted there, I belong there, it is my place on this earth. Here, like the many crows that crisscross the roads in front of us as we drive, I'm just passing through. I can check in with the land, discover things about it, marvel at the small magics I discover everywhere, but I don't *know* it the way I know the land of my birth.

In the book *The Mist-Filled Path,* the author recommends checking in with the guardians of each space you visit. Here now, in a hotel room in Nashville, Tennessee, I look out of the eighth floor picture window to note a series of five tree-covered hills to the right-hand horizon. They are clearly the sentinels of this valley city, I can see them watching, and I know that these are the guardians here.

At the roadside a billboard for coffee says something to the effect of, "because no one ever says they're too awake."

But, I think: *may we **all** be **too** awake.*

> *Be too awake.*
> *Trust the trembling forest*
> *place your hands on hot earth,*
> *on cold stones,*
> *in living streams.*
> *Look for bridges into mystery*
> *and thresholds into knowing*
> *formed of leaning trees*
> *and embracing roots.*

Be too awake
and let wings of wonder
carry you into clouds of magic
winding wisps of pleasure
through your blood
and bones.
Be too awake
and drink
all kinds of moonlight
curling yourself into caves
and groves
alive with meaning.
Be too awake
for the world
is full of birds
and you can feel the singing
in your soles
and skin.
Be too awake
for there are lakes of longing
within you
and you know how to swim.
Let the greening earth
glow beneath you
let your buried power
rise and breathe,
for it is in being too awake
that you will know yourself
as whole and here.
Be too awake
even if it is the only thing
you have left to be.

Careworn

We are home and it feels good. This morning my youngest child crawls into our bed and I feel my consciousness rising through layers of sleep, emerging from a world thick with dreams of visiting my extended family in California. I dreamed I was crying to my mother about how few people there are left to visit here. I wake thinking how this is true, how when I was a girl and we traveled to California, we would visit two sets of great-grandparents, two sets of grandparents and another great-grandmother. How we would see my aunts and uncle and cousins and my great-great Uncle Don. Now there is single great-uncle left, a step-grandfather, an aunt, an uncle, and a spattering of cousins, busy with their own families and lives.

This line of thinking leads me into dwelling on friendship and time and the evolving texture and terrain of friendships. How my time to tend to my friendships feels like it has dwindled with every year for the last fifteen years. How the richness of relationship fades without regular maintenance. How when I withdrew some of my own care and effort from the work of tending, the whole friendship faded to nothing, as if I were actually the only one holding it together, when I thought it was a reciprocal relationship.

I read some texts and Facebook conversations about this week's Pink Tent event. I find myself feeling like *I don't care*. I feel careworn, care-overloaded, care-burned out. Sometimes I even feel like I *can't* care anymore, like all my care is used up, spent, extinguished, exhausted. I'm a little sad and wistful thinking about how much I used to care, about everything, and I'm a little liberated by owning the "don't care" I feel in this moment. The world is stained, strained, and brittle from so much lack of care from so many people though. We *must* keep caring, we must care, even when it is a strain. I suppose the secret is not to care too much about things that don't require our care, not to overload ourselves with cares that are not our own, or that don't actually require our attention and are frankly, quite fine without us and our meddling.

I go to the woods. I sit on the rocks in the early sunlight, watching the way it glows through the small maple leaves, the dogwoods, the beginnings of the oak leaves. I hear a cacophony of blue jays. The wind bunches and curls, pushing into my back. I feel cold and disconnected, noticing the light in the leaves, but not really *feeling* it. I am distracted by thoughts and loss and ponderings on how much responsibility to hold and how much to release.

I feel alone and not in the sort of solitude I crave, but alone as if I have no one to ask for help if I needed it, alone as if unwanted. I feel like I need to recognize how I have pulled away from relationships with friends and extended family over the last several years, how my hunger for myself and for *time,* always more time, has led me to push them away, to be too busy for them. I do not want to be remembered as, or known for, being "too busy," and yet, I fear that is exactly the case.

I start to sing, *I am here,* in a low and throaty voice. I listen to the birds and watch the raspberry leaves and let myself feel the sensation of being alone.

I am here,
I am alive,
I am home,
all is well.

— Trina Brunk

The next morning, I wake with a knot of pain behind my eyes and also the awareness: *I am not a bad friend.* My self-recrimination on relationship-tending, while still raising questions that are important for any compassionate person to consider, is actually a symptom of a kind of pathological over-responsibility that I have struggled with since I was a teenager.

I think of my mother and my grandmother, both eldest daughters as well, and I can see this pattern in their lives as well. Always working to do it right, to please others, to perform admirably, to get it done, to do it well, and carrying resentment beneath the surface, about having to do it all, about always doing more and going above and beyond what anyone else will do. Isn't this the work of Air? Clearing out these patterns and thoughts, of cleansing away things that aren't working. These fears about being a bad friend that are rising up to haunt me immediately after returning home from two weeks on the road, caring for the lives and needs of six people, is actually part of a larger pattern — of never feeling like "enough" and of taking on more responsibility than needed for the experiences and feelings of others, as well as a common mental trick I use to hold myself down, shame myself, or otherwise berate myself for just being.

I am the eldest daughter of an eldest daughter of an eldest daughter. There are knots to undo.

What do you do with a careworn soul?
Do you let the threads continue
to thin and unravel
until you drift away
on a gossamer breeze?
Do you accept the numbness
of heart
that threatens to freeze
your hope?
Do you let the tears slip
down the back of your throat
and choke on unsung dreams?
Do you coil yourself down low
until you become poised to strike
and barbs grow on your tongue
and fingertips?
Or, do you let yourself cry
until you find yourself
awakening to a new day
and the wild violets are in bloom?
Do you spin the fibers
of your remaining love
into a cord of courage?
Do you gather seeds of almost forgotten dreams and nestle them
into the dark crevices that have formed
in your threadbare soul?
Do you find the cracks and holes
that have formed in your being
allow sunlight to peek around
the edges of yourself?
Do you let yourself become

soft and loamy
and feel the tender roots
of possibility winding down
into your bones
where you discover
something written on sinew
that feels like truth?

It is Time

I sit in the woods. The day is cloudy and gray again, but the small umbrellas of the maple leaves have opened wider. The rambunctious blue jays do not cease their calling and I see them swoop and argue, or court, over the branches of the oaks, laden with pollen and the green blush of newborn leaves. I miss the crows, those black birds have been an anchor for me during the last two weeks.

Persephone, please walk with me.

I feel the air curling around me insistently again, pushing on my back and shoulders. I am aware of a cool sensation, a tickle of air, right in front of my heart.

It is time.

To unwind the next loop from my soul.

I feel the cool spot of the lightly swirling breeze by my heart and I decide it is time to let the *pathological over-responsibility* blow away. Pathological over-responsibility, I whisper to the air swirling past my heart, *carry it away.* And then, no joke, a lone crow plummets into view from my right side, dropping silently in a rapid sweep into the valley and out of sight. I feel tears come to my eyes. I am so grateful. It feels nearly impossible to accept that I can be so heard, so held. But I see the evidence right before my eyes every single day and therefore it might be more impossible that these layers of life experiencing, of witnessing, are *not* connected, or that I am unheard.

I relax my arms and open my hands by my sides and just receive this gift of cleansing.

Loss

I wake thinking of my grandmother, Lyla. Yesterday was the sixth anniversary of her death. I still miss her and wish she was here. The dogwood blossoms are heavy with rain, nodding in their last stretch of glory before the greening of the woods closes in and the white petals fall. There are several more blooms on Noah's memorial magnolia tree, commemorating our third baby, who died in my second trimester.

The sky is heavy and gray again, but I feel a small swell of hope and peace when I stop by his tree and look at the flowers. I end up crying about my grandmother, the sensation of our time together having been cut unexpectedly short lingers. She left a hole in my life. I feel awash with emotions and also revisiting my own "lesson" about not needing to *fix anything*. I remind myself that it is okay to just let my feeling feel, to let my swoops swoop, to let my not-knowing not-know, to let my hope soar and then plummet, to let my joy be joyful, to let my tears be hot.

My grandmother's presence remains woven through my days: her quilt on my bed, a painting she loved on my kitchen wall, some of the dolls from her doll collection in my living room where I see them every morning and think of her.

I visited her Facebook page last night before bed feeling, as I always do, strange about the remnant of life preserved in this digital form — where it almost seems that something of her still lingers, present and observing. No wonder I feel weighty and sad. Her death was such a shock and her presence in our lives such a vibrant reality even though she lived 2,000 miles away.

After she died, I dreamed of her and she told me I would have seven dreams. In each dream, spaced widely apart, she would tell me how many dreams I had left. Finally, it was the last dream. There were in fact seven. And though I half think each April there will be another, there has not been.

Mist

The trees sing, the stones sing, the waters sing, the wind of the clouds sing, and the ancestors sing. Life is music. All things have their rhythm. The world is sound.

—Frank MacEowen, *The Mist-Filled Path*

I wake with my thoughts spinning and endlessly reviewing my to-do list, feeling thready, worn, and insubstantial, with a side dose of existential angst about the point of any of this. When I rise, though, I see mist curling through the woods and I taste mystery, potential, promise, a new story.

Everybody in the house is on edge, speaking sharply to each other, never-ending petty disputes over pointless topics.

I saw mist in the forest and it is whispering my name! I call to them and bypass the squabbling to step outside.

The leaves on the trees appear to have doubled in size overnight and the air is wet and green. I step down onto the mossy path into the woods, feeling a familiar and welcome tinge of excitement and anticipation, wonder and enchantment. It is as if I become enveloped in an alternate reality as I walk, stepping down and into this realm of presence and quiet. I pause at an overhanging hickory branch, feeling such anticipation about actually stepping into the mist, and then I cross the threshold onto the stones. I sit on a wet rock, feeling the rain from last night seeping into my jeans. The trees rise out of the mist, silently.

It is quiet and still. I feel like I am under a gray bowl. I feel like I am wrapped in a shroud. I feel like I am timeless, reborn, whole, and holy. This rock is the altar, the woods are the temple, the gray sky the cathedral. I find my mind scrabbling around for the right words, looking for the poem here in the tendrils of mist, in the silent witnessing. Finally, I give myself permission to just lay the words aside, remembering that some moments are meant to be held tenderly to the heart and don't need to be shared.

I don't need to try to remember or describe this, I just need to live into it, to feel my bones on the stones, my breath on my lips, my pulse in my wrist.

I close my eyes in this setting aside, letting my face soften, and feeling the sensation of being shrouded, held, enfolded, timeless, and then I hear the sound of a wild goose rising out of the mist. It rises, rises, rises, until it crosses overhead. Then, a wild chorus of crows break out at the unseen horizon line over the valley. I enjoy this sensation of foreshortened vision, of being contained rather than boundless, of having to rely on sound and not on sight, of sitting alone in a tiny, infinite misty world, enraptured, endless, enthralled.

Finally, I shake my head and blink several times, physically bringing myself back into my body and the awareness of the rest of the rhythms and needs of the day.

When I return to the house, it is like stepping out of one world and into another. What I wish for myself, for my family, is that the mist could always inhabit some corner of our knowing, our experiencing, rather than feel like an enchantment reserved for something other than "real life." This *is* real life and I'm glad I'm paying enough attention, sometimes, to step into it.

Hades and the Lake

When I finish teaching my co-op classes for the day, I follow the sounds of the red-winged blackbirds to the lake at the park across the street. The day is overcast and it is misting a little. There are two ducks on the lake, their lower halves streaked with green algae as they paddle along together. I pick my way through the mud and goose poop to my favorite tree, laden with pollen and new leaves, reaching out across the water, rising from a patch of wild violets.

I kneel in the violets, singing my Persephone song, feeling blissfully alone and renewed by this kiss of nature across my brow and beneath my fingers. I study the overhanging branches of the tree across the water and the way the raindrops sit on the violet leaves.

Suddenly, I look over my shoulder to discover I am not alone after all. There is a young man leaning against one of the tall cypress trees. He is not tall, dark, and Underworld, but rather sandy-haired, slight, and young enough to be my son, but I think of Persephone's tale anyway, especially since she has come to me so strongly here at this lake and now, here is Hades.

In the story of Persephone, she is gathering flowers in the meadows when Hades arrives to collect her, trailing Underworld shadows. Though I am nearly forty and far from Maiden as I squat in the violets, singing by a roadside lake in a Missouri town, I am still surprised to see an aspect of Persephone's story made flesh, walking out of time and onto the grass in front of me, leaning on one of the very same cypress trees in which I first heard her speak.

I decide to talk to him and tell him that I'm startled to see someone else there. He tells me he is there because it is the endpoint of his run and he stops here to enjoy the nature, this is his favorite place. I tell him it is one of mine too and then we bid each other good day. I head back to co-op and he remains, leaning on the tree, looking at the water, and watching the ducks. Despite feeling interrupted in my own personal experiencing, I also feel heartened to know that there are other people who find peace in this same spot and who value the stillness, the ripples of the water, and the tracks the ducks leave through the muck, just as I do.

We constantly weave life events into narrative and interpret everything that happens through the veil of story. From our smallest, most personal challenges to global issues that affect nations and generations, we make the world fit into the story we are already carrying. This unceasing interplay between experience and narrative is a uniquely human attribute. We are the storytellers, the ones who put life into words.

—**Christina Baldwin,** *Storycatcher*

Moonwise

I wake to bright sun streaming in the window and that knot of pain behind my eyes again. Some words from my mother last night keep rolling around my head: *you do seem to often be teetering at the brink.*

Something really stings for me here. Maybe instead of seeing me teetering at the brink, she could marvel at my capacity, at how very much I am handling, and doing, and being, and embodying, and living.

Can I even see that in myself though?

The only way I can actually see to stop teetering and to regain full footing, would be to withdraw *all* of my care work from almost all relationships, and that is not what anyone wants from me either. They actually want *more* caring, more time, more of my presence, not less. Never less. Just *one* more thing.

I think about how both my mother and my daughter would prefer my simple presence over anything: just spending time with me, and enjoying one another, but that I am always *doing* something instead, even if it is with them. I am rarely *just* present, because there is so much to do. The scraps of devotion that remain to me, I want to use on myself, on my own practices. *Didn't I also in some large part learn this from my mother? To do and do and try and try and work and work and then store up resentment within about not being appreciated enough or seen enough in all this striving and trying and providing and doing?*

This is it. I am here now. This is all that I have and all that I am. It isn't enough and yet it has to be, all in one.

Last night, we gathered in ritual for Pink Tent. This is the first ritual for which I haven't held primary responsibility for ten years. I still bring a carload of stuff, contributing significant supply resources to three of the four activity stations of the night. *What would have happened if I hadn't provided everything?* I wonder. I am responsible for painting pink moon magnets with the many, glowing, enthusiastic, wild little girls who attend. We weave flower crowns for ourselves, get mother-daughter portraits taken at sunset, sing around the fire, do a circle dance, feast and make merry. I barely see either my daughter or my mother, ironically, because there is so much activity and conversation and noise. I reflect on the drive home that in many ways our group has become too large to foster the kinds of experiences and relationships that it was originally meant to nurture. I'm not sure how to balance this—accessibility and community, with devotion, genuine connection and deep experience. My small solitary rituals and my simple family rituals hold more spiritual depth for me than a large, chattering, group experience and yet that is what I've built and cultivated and what continues to attract more and more interest.

During our ritual, the air is cold and the wind blows unpredictably and erratically. I watch a hawk circle as we sing and other birds that I don't recognize in firelit silhouette against the sky, but in many ways I feel disconnected, unmoored, buffeted by the thoughts, wishes, needs, and feelings of others, and fragmented, again, into so many unsustainable parts.

After we go inside to begin cleaning up, my mother, Barbara, calls us back outside, the full moon rising is finally visible over the treeline. Everyone hurries out the door and there she is! The full Pink Moon is on the rise, cresting the treetops, haloed with shades of orange and pink. She quickly moves past crowning and visibly moves upward in just a few minutes, a dramatic and sudden rise, rather than a slow and steady one. Each of us is enchanted by bearing witness to the rising. While it does happen every day, we are here, together in this moment, all noticing together. And we know we will never step into this moment twice. It is here, now, and then a new day will come and we will be different once more.

> *The world is full of dazzling maybes*[*]
> *let's make sure that it is also filled*
> *with dazzling living*
> *truths twined into being,*
> *prayers breathed into life,*
> *hope danced into blessing and blooming,*
> *and fairytales made flesh.*
> *If the opposite of wild,*
> *is tamed,*
> *let us never know*
> *that feeling on our skin.*
> *Let us braid flowers in our hair*
> *and sing below the moon,*
> *spinning poems*
> *alive beneath a fierce*
> *and open sky.*

[*] "Dazzling maybe" inspired by the book *Silverswift*, by Natalie Lloyd

The Lying Down Revolution

In the woods now this morning, sitting on the stones, and watching the light filter through the maple leaves, it is almost impossible to hang on to my disillusionment and worn, tiresome questioning. Maybe I could *thank* my sensation of wanting to let go of caring, because it shows me how much and how deeply I have cared. Maybe I can thank the sensation of trying too hard as wanting to do my best work and live up to my potential. Maybe I can stroke the agitation of doing too much with soft fingers of understanding and acknowledgment that trying to do too much is a symptom and sign of having a full and vibrant life and a reminder of how very much good work there is to do in the world, so much purpose that calls my name. How fortunate I am to be so full, to be attached to so many people and causes and projects, these things are signs, the symptoms, and the threads of a vibrant life of deep care and a wellspring of love. There is no shame needed in offering out what you have within you to give and there is no shame in stepping back and saying, *enough*.

At the ritual last night, a friend tells me that she has been going to yoga class and every time she lies on the floor at the end of class, she thinks of me. I consider this a compliment. If I could be known as a lying-down revolutionary, that would please me. At least two years ago, I put on my "100 Things to Do this Year" list, to lie on the floor for at least three minutes every day. I have kept this up more or less every day since then, even setting my phone timer for three minutes at the end of my personal yoga practice each morning, so I know I'm actually giving this to myself.

What might change for many of us if we allowed ourselves three minutes a day to lie on the floor? Ten minutes? Fifteen minutes? One hour? Another friend tells me she needs a time out to refill herself until she is overflowing, instead of just refilling her cup a tiny bit and then draining it over and over again. I feel this too. I have been coasting on my reserve tank for at least a year and my reserves are now depleted too. It takes more than three minutes to fill the tank so that it has sustained and lasting energy to fuel my soul.

I sit with my eyes closed in the sunshine, basking in the warmth. I hear the sound of birds from each side of me, ping-ponging off of one another into the sparkling green air. I listen to them until my mind softens and I am no longer tormenting myself with questions of how to be better, be more, fix it. I am very still on the rock and when I open my eyes, I see a vulture coasting towards me. It swoops, possibly checking to see if I am actually breathing there on the stone. It circles once, twice, three times, above my head, at each pass coming low enough that I can see its red head turn from side to side, looking at me. *Hey, buddy,* I say. *Yes, I'm still breathing!*

My floor-lying friend has spent the night at my parents' lodge and I go to visit her and to paint with my mom, my daughter, and my friend and her family. My head still throbs with pain and I don't feel very present, but we paint anyway, the colors swirling and mixing and the freeform nature of the pour painting meaning there are no mistakes, only magic. I help her load a weaving loom into her car and we speak briefly about group dynamics and ritual etiquette, and priestessing energetics. As we speak, I look up to see nine vultures this time, circling in the wide sky above the large open field surrounding the lodge building. They dance in the air and they whisper: *It is okay to let go. It is okay to soar. It is okay to be free. It is okay to clean it out and away.*

> *Sometimes I feel like my work—*
> *for others and for myself—*
> *is about calling us back*
> *into our bodies,*
> *edges both strong and soft,*
> *about calling ourselves*
> *back into our own lives,*
> *both small enough*
> *and big enough*
> *to hold who we are.*
> *Ceremonies of bones and skin,*
> *prayers of salt and tears,*
> *rituals of mud and sun,*
> *a sacred story of body*
> *and breath*
> *and being*
> *in the world*
> *as it unfolds*
> *beneath our feet.*

After painting, I come home to our still-trashed house after our trip. The suitcases haven't been unpacked, there are piles of unfolded laundry, the kids have decided to excavate old toys from the closet and the couch cushions are all on the floor. I also still haven't taken the product photos I've been meaning to take for days. And the back of my car is still filled with Pink Tent supplies.

When I get to the deck, I realize that I'd really like to just lie down for a while in the sun and so I lie flat on my back, with my eyes closed, my arms open at my sides, thinking of my lying on the floor revolution. I find myself drifting into a sort of half-conscious trance and it is the most delicious sensation. It is warm, the birds are singing, I feel held and grounded, and like I've called my spirit back into my body.

I am like this for at least an hour, and when I finally sit up again, I feel restored. I draw my card from Womanrunes and receive, no joke, The Sun, rune of healing.

Mark has joined me outside and is sleeping in the porch swing. I stand by the deck rail and see a swoop of black and white. I think it is a woodpecker at first, perching on a nearby oak, but then I recognize it as something else. It is black and white with a red spot on its breast. It is a rose-breasted grosbeak! The first one I remember ever seeing.

I Am Open

I wake to a bright shaft of sunlight in the room, the cry of a hawk on the wind, and the lyrics from the song "My Soul" by Suzanne Sterling and Jeffrey Mooney replaying in my head. *I am breathing, I am open, I am willing.*

I receive a question from a customer asking me about the structure of my poems, *what do I call the style in which I write them?* I have too many thoughts for an email, so I make an audio recording that explores the complex and multifaceted terrain of this question.

It is almost as if the poem is happening, I explain, and I've stepped up to it and I've seen it and then I write about it. The poem is there, in the world, in the moment, and all I do is write it down.

That requires:

Showing up…to witness

A quietness…to listen

A willingness to be active, to participate, in the hum of creation.

I will sit in the woods and I will feel the poem, I will see the story, I will hear a phrase, and the poem shapes itself into being from that.

While I make my audio recording, sitting on the porch of the tiny temple, I watch two hummingbirds visit first the tulips and then the hummingbird feeders. I see a vulture soar by in front of me *right* as I tell the story of saying "I'm still breathing" to the vulture above me in the woods just the other day. I continue to hear the hawk call, insistently, crying out repetitively. I step out under the sky several times to look for it, but only hear the sounds. Finally, I walk to the back deck, where it disappears from sight. But I can still hear it.

I feel like I'm supposed to learn something, to listen, to respond. So I stand in the dandelions and violets in front of the tiny temple, staring up into the bright blue sky. I see the hawk, high in the air above me. Suddenly it drops lower and lower, so it is just skimming the treetops and *then* it flies directly over the house, so low it is only about one foot above the shingles. As I stare, transfixed and almost shaking with wonder, it lands right in the oak tree across from me. I stand motionless, staring at it, feeling a visual, tunneling effect in which the surrounding area becomes blurred and only the hawk is in focus.

I feel tears in my eyes, I feel wonder that this is even possible, that it is even happening, that I am watching a new poem unfold in front of my eyes, right after speaking of exactly this. *This is the magical world I live in. It is real and it is right here.* I look up and see a second hawk, still high in the air. It sweeps away into the woods past the hawk sitting in the tree, who then flies off to join it.

Animism is a way of experiencing life so that we are constantly awakened to the preciousness of our moments on this earth. While not a religion per se, animism is an informed spirituality characterized by handing oneself over to the authentic, untainted experience of the universe from the vantage point of sacred eyes, sacred senses, and an open heart.

—Frank MacEowen, *The Mist-Filled Path*

I sit in silence staring and thinking about poems, how they find me, how I walk up to or into them, how I rarely write a poem out of anything but direct experience — something I've actually seen that very day. I do not create metaphors out of them (usually) or make them into stories or lessons that aren't already there, waiting for me. I don't make up pieces that would sound good or invent animals that weren't present because they'd tie it together better. The poems just happen and I see them. I am so still and absorbed in thought that when I finally swallow, the sound of it startles me.

The Ninth Task

After a hazy night of whirling dreams, I wake to clear, bright blue skies, and sunlight streaming in the window again. I am tired. Tired of being tiresome, of making the same complaints, of spinning my wheels in the same way, of being stuck in the same patterns. I've made some changes this year that are good, but I feel like many of my lessons are not sticking: I have to keep learning them.

I decide I should print them on a little card and carry them around. Having insights is one thing, *doing it* is another thing. At the same time, I wonder how much "fixing" of my personality I truly need to do. Maybe I can just soften into it? Maybe one of the things I am learning is simply that there is an ebb and flow to my mood, my feelings, my level of enchantment, just as some days are sunny and some are raining and some are mist-ical.

> *The ninth task*
> *is to embrace*
> *the ebb and flow*
> *of life and being.*

There is no fixing needed.

In the woods, I sit on the cool, damp stones. The trees to my left are glowing in the still-young sun of the day, the edges of each leaf sparkling with freshness and possibility. The sky is blue and the breeze curls around my arms, on the very edge of too cold. A fallen oak supported by two comrades still alive creaks and groans in an ominous way. I am thinking about how I am restless and feeling eager to move on to the next phase of my journey, I keep wondering about which goddess I will work with next, about the element I will explore. I think about the lessons so far and my sense that they are not sticking, that there is more work left to do. But, then I think of Hades in the flowers by the lake, and my dream of walking through the corridor of death last night, *you cannot make this stuff up*, I think, *Persephone is not through with me yet.* And right as I think that, right as I know with such certainty that she is not done with me yet, a vulture rises out of the trees and flies past me on quiet wings.

May you follow your longing
right up to the heart of your living
and find it is here
right now.

The List

It is raining heavily this morning, so I spend time coloring letters to fairies with the children and writing a list of the things I need to refuel my soul and restore my care so that I can be there for others, for our work. My list is simple and short.

1. Go to the woods.

2. Write and journal.

3. Walk and discover things.

4. Create/draw/take pictures.

5. Read.

Mark points out that I actually do the things on it almost every day.

I realize I reserve these special, sacred, soul-fueling moments for the beginnings and endings of each day. My days are bookended by magic moments — my mornings in the woods, my evenings on our walks—but, the centers can feel dry, parched, and pushy. I wonder if the bookends are enough, or if I need to consciously shift even more into the center of my days.

When I finally do go to the woods, it is afternoon, the rain has stopped, the day has become warm and the clouds are white and puffy in a blue sky. Two of my kids follow me, talking in loud voices that interrupt my peace and add to the pulse of pain in my head.

I watch a white butterfly dance around the leaves and then a blue butterfly. I hear the hawk. I answer the kids' questions. The breeze is busy and swirls around me. I remember that caring, that showing up, that being present, includes *this too,* it isn't reserved only for small slices of solitary, magic moments of connection with the Goddess and inner peace, it is being here with my headache, with my noisy, excited, loving children, it is continuing to care when I feel worn and fragile, because caring is what holds life together.

This is the wildness
that sustains me.
This is the witnessing
that strengthens me.
This is the wonder
that softens me.

A Whole-Assed Life

I wake from the middle of dreams to the abrupt sound of three loud taps on my bedroom window. Even though nothing is actually there. This happens sometimes, when I've overslept, like an internal alarm system.

I feel a soft squish of blood between my legs and remember, as I often do, that despite how body-honoring I am, despite how immersed in Red Tent work I am, the trend my thoughts take towards despair, burnout, dissatisfaction, frustration, occurs on a regular, reliable, and predictable pattern each month. I do not ever like to blame hormones for genuine frustrations, for problems in living and relationships that are easier to stuff down and ignore when my endocrine system is more robust, but that bubble upward into tears and tantrums when my hormones take a dive. It isn't "not real" to be upset about something that agitates at me at some level all month, but that I don't allow to escape in words until I am worn, frayed, tired, and depleted, and only then do they surface, angry and denied. At the same time, I can also recognize a fog that descends and then lifts each month like a wave or a tidal rhythm.

The closing lines from my "Too Awake" poem are playing and replaying through my head so insistently that I almost can't finish my morning prayers:

It is in being too awake that you will know yourself as whole and here.

I see two crows flying by along the horizon line and step out of the door into surprisingly cold air, with a sense of anticipation. There is a red cardinal on a dogwood tree amongst the white flowers. His mate is picking through the leaves at the base of the tree, intent. I sit on the stones listening and feeling encased in sound. The thick green leaves make it hard to see very much now and instead of feeling enraptured by a sweeping vista, I feel cocooned in a green bubble, a hollow in the palm of the forest, where it is my ears that need to become sharp and not my eyes. I notice many whirling thoughts chattering by: of friends, the mysteries of their marriages and why they stay, cooking pork loin for family potluck tonight, what to wear to a tea party today... They swirl and dip and dance.

I become aware of the air, cool, insistent, bumping against my head, and I soften. I feel the sensation again of the top of my head being open and I let the cool air sweep away all these thoughts, whisk me clean. I turn to see three blue jays fly up and alight in the tree. They fly back and forth between several trees, talking and fluttering. I am silent and small on the rock below, watching. I turn back from the jays just in time to see three vultures rising from the valley and catching the air above the tree not far from me. While there is nothing specifically powerful happening, I feel captivated, curled in this cocoon of green and sound.

I think about how sitting on a rock in the same place every day *changes everything*. I know where the sound of the mourning doves will rise each morning, I know where the wild turkeys wander and gobble for their breakfasts, I know the routes the crows take across the sky, and I know how the vultures like to dance over this valley. It is magical to know your place, to know yourself as entwined with the rhythms and habits and habitats of innumerable other lives, to become small under a broad sky, to become still on a cold rock, to forget to swallow with the intensity and presence of it all, right here, right now.

I am wondering why it is that I only, or most often, feel *whole* when I'm alone. *Why do I only truly like myself when I'm solitary, or alone as a self-sovereign human with just Mark or just one other adult?* I often do not feel like a good parent, I feel splintered and split by parenting, I feel edgy and sharp and distracted. I am feeling tense and unhappy about having agreed to go anywhere today, because I could really have used the time to just focus on being *here*, to work on my journals, to lie in the sun, to spend some time simply breathing and being. But, I don't want to let down my friend and I also relish the idea of some friendship time just on my own.

I shower with my two youngest children in with me so they can get their hair washed. I am constantly wracked with the fear that I'm not doing "enough" for them, that I'm not available enough, present enough, connected enough, enjoying them enough, *being* enough for them. It is one of the most crippling shadows in my adult life, worrying that I am failing my kids, that they will remember me as unhappy, distracted, maxed out, stressed, and sad.

I dress in my red renaissance faire dress and put on my flower crown from Pink Tent and go to my friend's costume tea party. While there, we turn over the bonds and restrictions in our lives in an intense and often vulnerable conversation. As we talk, I watch a blue jay land on her deck. In telling them how I always want to give things my best effort, I find myself describing myself as a "whole-assed person."

I do things with my whole ass, I say, *I live a whole-assed life and that is okay with me.* And it is. But I'm not always capable of putting my whole ass into things, even if I want to, even if I know that is how I do my best work, because there is always someone else who needs me and that is one of the restrictions that chafes the most.

In my conversation with my friends we also talk about happiness and meaning and *what is the point, anyway?* I assert that I think we have a choice in life, to see everything as having meaning or nothing as having meaning, and I choose the first. I also know that it isn't reasonable to expect to feel happy all the time. *How can we recognize happiness without some counterpoint emotional experiences? But, if we are just going through the motions of our lives, if we are feeling hollow and dull and extinguished, instead of happy, then truly, what is the point?*

The lesson I know I have not yet learned from Persephone is the difference between choice and force. I feel "forced" in life more often than I would like—forced by myself, ironically, most often and forced by needs of others. I often feel pushed and driven by *something* other than my own free will. I have determined that I will journey into the Underworld of unraveling and rebuilding my soul by choice, not by force, knowing that if I do not choose it my body or spirit will force me to take the journey.

What would it feel like to truly be guided by active choice in my days, rather than self-imposed or environmental force?

What if I abandoned the use of force on my own spirit?

What if I became unwilling to force, but just sat on a rock with my hands open, waiting to know?

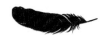

Sometimes you'll arrive
at the changing edges
of an uncertain world,
your life in your hands,
wondering what to do.
Sometimes you'll arrive
at the tender edges
of your own life,
dreams in your eyes,
prayers in your feet,
magic in your blood,
fire in your belly,
and art in your hands.
Sometimes you'll journey
from the edges of uncertainty
back to the center
where you'll find a garden
tended neat and nourishing
or unkempt and flourishing.
Sometimes you'll discover

you've made everything harder
than it needs to be.
Sometimes you'll lean in
to see that it can be
easier than you think,
to love your edges,
to live your limits,
to tend the garden
where you grow best,
wild, rambling
and rich with dirt and flowers.

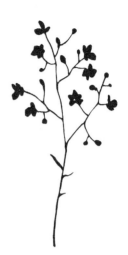

MAY

May Day

The first morning of May dawns heavy, green and gray. The ground is saturated from the heavy rainfall last night and the trees are drooping under the avalanche of water. I step outside wondering again about next steps. *Is what I'm doing making any sense? How do I know what to do next? Where to go next? Whether anything is actually "working?"* As I step along the mossy stones to the woods, ducking under wet, low-lying branches, I hear:

Keep walking. Keep seeing.

Is that enough though? How will I know what to do? I can hear the rushing sounds of the flooded creek from here, though it is down the hill and in the valley, far out of sight. I sprinkle a circle of hawthorn leaves and jasmine flowers around the stone on which I sit and swipe the first May dewdrops off the hickory tree to anoint my forehead, eyes, lips, throat, heart, belly, hands, and feet, offering gratitude and love to myself for being right here right now.

Persephone, I whisper, *I need to know the next steps…please give me a sign.*

Before I can finish my sentence, as the words "a sign" are actually on my lips, a crow flies from the woods and over my shoulder.

Keep walking. Keep seeing.

I am two days away from turning forty. I sit on the wet stone, letting the water seep into my pants, surrounded by hawthorn and raindrops. I am encircled by magic. I am alive with meaning. I am hopeful. I am whole.

I am encircled by magic.

I feel held by my circle of herbs, the green trees, the mystery of this May morning. The sound of a hawk, red-tailed this time, rises out of the valley, insistent and strong. It rises and rises, finally tracing an audible line from the horizon to a tree to my right, where it pauses. I do not see it, though that would be even more magical, and then with a cry, it takes off again and continues, the sound dying away finally over the field in front of the house as it passes out of my range.

Forty

It is my fortieth birthday and I wake early to a darkening, rain-laden sky. I was born on a rainy morning and rain on my birthday, which often happens, feels like a birthday greeting from the land, to me: *you still belong here.*

I feel anticipatory, but also on the verge of tears: delicate, fragile, friable.

In the woods, the path is carpeted with white flower petals as the dogwoods drop their blooms, and I sit on the stone with my arms wrapped around my legs wondering what I will experience, receive or learn today. I hear the soft, insistent cooing of the mourning doves, deep within the woods. The wind picks up and sweeps the top of my head, with a cool feeling I recognize. *What will I surrender today? Which knot will I untie?*

I decide that in honor of my birthday I will give myself the gift of letting go of not being good enough. This is different than not being *enough*, it is intimately entwined with "good-ness" and it has shadowed me for so long that it feels it is almost an intrinsic part of me. As soon as I decide that it can go, the distant sound of a barred owl drifts up from the hollow.

I am not sure what I am expecting, but I thought it would be easier. First, I let myself feel the sensation fully, really washing over me, settling in: *not good enough.* Then, after it has washed through my body, I let the wind start to sweep it away. I feel the coils of the not-good-enough sensation unraveling from inside, detaching from the plains of my mind.

But once detangled, it does not want to lift. I close my eyes and see it rising above my head and think, *now, I should cut it off.* However, I see that if I cut, the root of it remains, still twined deep in my brain, still there. Only the surface feeling is rising, the root remains. I must loosen the root too. It is white and thick and branched and it is settled there, in my brain. I think of how people cut cords, battle demons, excise wounds. I think of banishing, I think of tugging, I think of uprooting, I think of exploding, I think of extracting, but none of these are right. I need to let the feeling soften, tenderize, rise, and float. I need to let it gently, gently separate.

This could take a long time, I know.

I look up to see a crow on silent wings swoop directly over my head.

I let my eyes drift back closed and continue to sit, feeling increasingly intense sensations in my head and body. I feel like my brain is rippling and squeezing, like it is quivering and vibrating, I feel an almost orgasmic sensation of contraction and release sweeping through my head over and over. I see the white root loosen and rise until only a tendril remains connected at the top back of my skull, where my fontanel would have been as a newborn. The tendril remains stuck there, connected, the rest of the white mass is tethered to my skull by a delicate strand. I open my eyes to see two more crows, noisy ones, passing by along the treeline. I try to send the feeling with the crows, but it doesn't want to go. I again think of cutting, but I want it to detach on its own.

I close my eyes again and continue to feel waves of sensation and then I realize, I am afraid to let it go. There are small fingers within me that are reaching up to it, trying to pull it back down, grasping and struggling to hold it in place, to keep connected to this feeling I have held for so long.

I'm not ready for it to leave me. I don't know who I will be when it is gone.

I continue to wait, feeling the sweeping breeze, the contraction and release inside my skull. *I will know,* I tell myself, *I will know.* I can't force it before it is ready to go. A buzz surprises me, and I open my eyes to see a female humming-bird in the air right in front of me, investigating my presence. The sound of her wings is loud and I immediately feel the sensation that the plates of my skull have slid back together, snapped shut like a lid. *Ah ha!* I think, *this is my sign, the closing of my skull will have severed the tendril.* I even sweep my hand over my head to try to shake the tendril away. But it is still there. I can feel it. The shape has changed, so I have the sensation that it is the small toe of a little creature that is caught there, one toe of the feeling still anchored within me.

It is okay, I say. *Thanks for trying so hard to always keep me safe. You've done enough.* I want to stay outside, stay with the process, but it is time to go in and so I do, reluctantly. I tell myself I've let the feeling go, that it has unwound and been set free, but whenever I check, it is still there, bobbing at the end of this tether at the back of my skull. I carry it through the morning, my awareness so physical and real, I almost feel like other people surely see this white shadow, barely connected to me, bobbing along above the top of my head.

I take our two youngest children to my parents' house. Two iris flowers the color of rust have bloomed in front of the house and my mom takes my picture by her huge snowball bush. *How am I forty?* we wonder together. I see how this is middle-aged—in this liminal space between youth and age. I could be at the exact midpoint of my lifespan. My mom tells me that I changed her whole world, that I changed the world of everyone in the family: her parents, my aunt and uncle, everything was rocked by my entry into this life. *I promoted you all,* I laugh, *you all leveled up because of me.* We both cry then, embracing by the rain-dappled iris blooms.

Perhaps, I think as I drive away, *it really is possible that I am truly loved.* The white specter of not-good-enoughness bobs quietly above my head.

At home, I print some more orders, give some more instructions, and the morning continues to slip away. Mark packs me a little lunch bag and fills my water bottle and I declare that I am setting out on my adventure. I take the long way to the river, due to a flooded road.

A turtle crosses the road in front of me. Next, three vultures rise up from the road. And then a crow passes in front of me.

I have taken bags of art supplies, decks of oracle cards, and mounds of journals with me to the river, but as soon as I arrive, I know I only want to walk. The wild white violets are in bloom. I hear crows out of sight and the rush of the flooded water. I find the tiny half of an eggshell.

As I walk by the creek, three vultures soar above me and I feel a tug on the cord connecting me to my separating shadow feeling. She—it has come to be clearly female now, and winged—is considering going with the vultures. *You can go with them,* I say, and the cord separates. She tries to fly with them, but they wheel and disappear, and she is left hovering in the air above my head, no longer connected, but lingering nearby. *Thank you,* I say, *I love you. You can go.*

As I watch her try several small flights I realize, *What will I do without you? Who will I be?* Her wings aren't strong enough to carry her away and so I continue my walk as she flies along behind me. I see a black and white striped butterfly with some red spots and I wonder if my little good-enoughness fairy wants to fly away with it, but she doesn't.

I tiptoe over murky underbrush, flattened by floodwater, and duck under heavy limbs, pushing past quickly overgrown bushes and plants. I see trillium and Jack-in-the-pulpit and a meadow of mayapples. I see that the wild geraniums are in bloom. As I make my way along the barely visible path, I find a raccoon skull sitting solemnly in the branches of a tree. I laugh with delight to see it, thinking how amazing it is that you cannot make this stuff up. Go for a walk on my birthday, find a skull in a tree. It feels perfect.

I carry the skull on the rest of my journey, up steep banks and slippery mud dotted with deer hoof prints, teetering across mossy stones, and past wildflowers. As I emerge from the underbrush by the big spring, I see a mother duck and thirteen ducklings swimming in the spring. The mother flies away, startled, and leaves all of the babies, milling about in small circles. They are tiny and vulnerable and I am entranced by them. It feels like the best birthday present of my life.

As I make my way back along the sodden path, I stop by a small cave to photograph a goddess in the wild geraniums, one of my favorite spring flowers. I am thinking about life as I squat to take my pictures and I wonder briefly if I am trying too hard to *make* my life be magical, be meaningful. And then I realize,

If you look for evidence that the world is made of magic, for evidence that your life is magical, you will find it everywhere.

This isn't wrong. This isn't tricking myself. This is beautiful and powerful and real. Yes, my life is magical. The whole world is magical. We need only step right up to it and look, to see that we are surrounded by magic, woven right into the threads of it.

Back in the field by the cabin, I settle on the porch to eat my little picnic. I look over to see a lone vulture approaching. It circles lazily and I sense the little white fairy yearning in its direction. *It's okay,* I tell her, *you can go.* The vulture comes closer and the fairy flies up to it. The little cord is gone now, she just has wings. They fly together and I watch them swoop and dip on the currents of air. They rise higher, further from me, dipping over the trees. I sense her looking back at me and I suddenly know:

You can go, I tell her, *I'll be okay without you.*

And, as I blow her a kiss, they both drop out of sight behind the trees.

As I typed this story on the porch of the river cabin, a female hummingbird flew down directly in front of me and hovered, staring at me.

What If?

I open my eyes this morning to a hummingbird hovering outside the bedroom window looking in.

While the day dawns with a sense of possibility, I am quickly weighed down with responsibilities, oddly neglecting my own practice of going to the woods immediately and instead focusing on "getting a few things done," before I go.

The few things quickly turn into afternoon. Our youngest child develops a fever and a stomachache. And I find myself at 2p.m. still waiting to do yoga and journal in preparation to start the day. I always look forward to long days at home with no employees at work and nowhere to go. But with no defined structure to the day, no outside forces to shape it, and many conflicting needs of many different family members with different ideas of what constitutes an ideal "day off," days with no imposed, external structure can easily become blobby, amorphous, full of never-ending, neglected minutiae and catch-up.

Finally, I drag myself away from the computer and go to the woods for a few minutes. As always, I feel a welcome peace descend. The sky is light gray, almost white today. I see a black and white spider with incredibly long legs nestled in the hollow of a leaf. The maple leaves are fully spread open now, the landscape and visibility further sunken into a realm of endless green. I hear an odd noise and see a brown bird I don't recognize flitting about near the ground and into the cedar trees. It makes a sound I can't identify, harsh and croaky. I feel droopy and dreary. Closed in and weary. I notice that now that my birthday has passed I also feel a sensation of relief or release. Anticipating the milestone of forty has perhaps been weighing on me more than I knew, a sensation of unacknowledged "deadline" and pressure that is now relieved.

What if you have all the time you need?
I wonder, as I watch the mysterious brown bird.
What if there is no need to force,
what if it can all come easy?
What if you are truly loved?
I lie on my back on the cold stone. The air has a tinge of chill and I have worn a sweater. I curl my knees into my chest and close my eyes. I feel drifty, tired, uncertain and before I know it, my legs drop a bit and I think I may have been slipping off into sleep. I feel disoriented and stale. I've noticed this before—an intensity of spiritual experience, an awakening, a magical experience, a real-life

journey, a significant ritual, a personal initiation, may be followed the subsequent day by a type of ennui, staleness, frustration, and confusion, as if life is not, in fact, magical enough for me after all, or as if I'm waiting for something to "top" the experience of the day before.

Your Work

I wake from a dream in which I received a message about the wings of an eagle. But like an eagle in flight, the message slips from my memory as I open my eyes to bright sun glittering through the rain-spangled trees.

I am thinking about how the rhythm of my days has changed over the last five years. How I used to rely on my "two hours" to rebuild my soul almost every day and how now those two-hour blocks are scant to none, save Mondays when I am alone all day, usually working feverishly in an attempt to do a week's worth of work in my single, solitary day. No wonder I often feel taut and faded, with crumbling edges.

My mind is slippery today, skipping around from reflection to judgment to memory to evaluation to assessment to criticism to wondering to appreciation. I watch each type of thought flitter around and instead of feeling disappointed in myself for not being able to calmly settle, I feel humbled with gratitude for having such an active, beautiful, complex brain that can think in so many ways. When gratitude enters, conflict dissolves.

I am thinking about work and how I feel a tension or imbalance between what our business asks of us, the work tasks I need to complete, and what I need to feel whole, healthy, and in balance within myself.

Your work itself is vital. Doing your work is living this path. Being here right now is part of your work.

I think about meaning and making meaning and how many people have told me that our work, my art, our little goddess sculptures, add meaning to their lives. Some people feel like life has no meaning, but I feel like meaning is woven throughout everything I do. Looking out into the filtered light in the maple leaves, I can see the weaving right in front of my eyes. If these goddess figures we make give people something to hold on to, that reminds them of their thread in this weaving, that connects them physically, emotionally, spiritually to the Goddess and to goddess paths and ways of being, I have done my job.

How can I bring more mindfulness and intention to the tasks that feel rote and boring though? How can I sprinkle more magic and connection into the center of my days instead of bookending my self-created grind with morning and evening dollops of magical living?

I need more pauses, more opportunities to lie on the floor, more micro-adventures, more discoveries.

I go to the tiny temple to collect some supplies for Red Tent and pause to take a photo of one of my She Listens goddesses by a triplet of oak leaves glittering with raindrops. As I do, a message floats to mind:

> *Reminder:*
> *You are not one long, relentless*
> *self-improvement project.*
> *You are a marvel of art and fire*
> *and the world is in your eyes.*

I am setting everything aside and I'm going to see what is left.

Walking with the Goddess

This morning I open *Aspecting the Goddess* by Jane Meredith. I've gotten through the chapter about Persephone before, but it was earlier this year and I feel like I will have better continuity and context if I read it again in earnest from the beginning.

Jane describes one way of studying and working with specific goddesses as "walking with," writing:

> *Walking with a goddess is a way of granting us some insight into her myths or stories. Walking with can be an introduction to a goddess we don't know, perhaps one who has appeared in a dream or whose name has leapt out at us...*

I remember how my original breath of a prayer, *Persephone, please walk with me,* came to me so clearly and I am curious and intrigued to watch myself continue to deepen into my exploration in this way. It *is* a walk together. I like the active component implied by the word *walk,* I like the sensation of intent and purpose as well as companionship. It is also a listening.

In my intuitive understanding of what it is to *walk with* a goddess, it means dipping deep into her story as a living experience of moving through the world. Bringing her story, symbols, and experiences into your own life, of considering yourself *accompanied*. It means to move through your days, through your being, your actions and choices as if you are in contact with and relationship with the goddess herself—alert for symbols, signs and connections that bring the magical into the mundane. It is not a subservient relationship, or even a devotional relationship, and not a ministerial relationship, but a companionable relationship, a sensation and reality of moving through the world, through your own life and story, inspired, guided by, and accompanied by a divine presence, guidance, or perhaps simply the inspiration and encouragement you have drawn from the stories of the past. Walking with a goddess can be about getting to know her, about deepening into her, about weaving an understanding of how her story, values, experiences, and symbols intersect with your own.

Mother's Day

It is Mother's Day, but it is also the twenty-fourth anniversary of our first date: a first (and last) first date experience for either of us. Mark asked me out as we took a walk together at the park, after coming to my surprise sixteenth birthday party the day before. On our first date, we went for a walk at a different park. We have walked together almost every evening for the last twenty-four years, whether we lived in a small apartment in the city or in the middle of the woods. People sometimes ask for our "secret" and it might just be found on our walks.

We've walked carrying toddlers, pushing strollers, and at forty weeks pregnant. We've walked around our back deck when it was too dark to walk anywhere else. We've even walked in circles in the living room and kitchen when it is snowing. We've walked with kids between us and we've walked holding hands. We've walked on the beach, in mountains, by rivers, across fields, in mud and in rain. On Mother's Day today, the gift I asked for was to go on a walk in the woods.

These woods endlessly replenish my spirit and nourish my soul and sense of being. I stop to take a picture in the blackberry blossoms of my oracle cards of the day and a tiny mother-daughter goddess charm. The flowers are glittering with captured raindrops in some shafts of brave sunlight that are managing to creep from behind still more gray clouds. As I kneel carefully in the blackberries, a shadow of wings crosses me and I look up to see a vulture, circling over the roof, the deck, my head. It is close enough for me to see the sun reflecting off the white pattern on the underside of its wing tips. I tip my head back to watch it, smiling.

I cannot believe I was withholding this from myself. It is right here.

If there is anything I could communicate with or share with anyone, it is this magic, this connection with the soul of place. This engagement with what *is*. This stepping out and into what is right *here,* waiting. Or, not waiting, as the case may be, existing whether or not we pause to pay attention, solace dripping from it like raindrops off blackberry.

We clamber over the wet, mossy trunks of fallen trees and examine the thick cords of knotted roots lacing their way under the stony creek bed. This is what I needed and wanted most of all today, not a clean house or breakfast in bed, but to marvel at roots and stones. I tell Mark that I'm worried that people will think I'm saying that all anyone needs to fix their problems is to sit on a rock in the woods. But then I realize that *is* kind of what I am saying! Not everyone has a rock or the woods though, so I am an advocate for finding the soul of place wherever you are, whether in a backyard, a neighborhood park, a state park, or even a slice of treeline you can see from a balcony and get to know the birds.

I finally finished reading Frank MacEowen's book, *The Mist-Filled Path,* which I started at the beach in January. He concludes it with this wish:

May you find your resurrection place, your own forest shrines, and trust that what you discover there is good. May you come to embrace the wisdom the mist can teach us about blending, about making compromises in our fixed and solidified states of mind, and may you learn to trust and rely on the holiness of the longing in your soul.

I have found my resurrection place, I know my forest shrine, and I am trusting the holiness of the longing in my soul.

It is from this book that I also read of the concept of "place-bonding" for the first time that I can remember, even though I've taken graduate level coursework in ecopsychology and write from an eco-psychological perspective. This refers to forming an emotional, heart-connection to an environmental location, similar to pair-bonding with another human, the bond of love is formed between a human and her place.

If this is wonder,
I'll share it,
because it is wondering
that we wander into ourselves.
If this is mystery,
I'll hold it,
because deep inside,
the mystery waving back
tells me it is what weaves
this world together.
If this is wisdom,
I'll whisper it,
for the world
is full of voices,
waiting to be heard.

A Crisis of Abundance

As I lie on my yoga mat in *savasana,* it comes to me, another task for gentling my days:

Witnessing without fixing.

This thought feels like a deep, nourishing, exhale.

I think of a poem I wrote several weeks ago about not sharing everything. I'm noticing an increasing pressure within myself of needing to make sure I have "enough" inspirational things to share on social media. I've been reflecting on my own relationship with myself, with my wisdom, with my truths, with my heart, with that which I need to know, do, or write for *myself* and not for the consumption of others. And this means that I can write poems I don't share. I can have thoughts I don't record. I can have insights I don't teach.

You do not have to give
everything away
or share every scrap
of insight
in order to be real.

You can nestle some
stories
and some silence
right under your breast,
shh, shh, it's okay.
Drink deeply of life
and what you have made from it.
This is your weaving.
This is your blood.
This is your pain.
This is your truth.
This is your song.
Remember to keep singing.

My friend comes to pick up her son who has been spending the night with my older boys and we go for a short walk first. As we stroll down the gravel road under the bright sunshine and into the humid air, we talk briefly about our full to bursting lives. I tell her about my theory of a "crisis of abundance," and note that my life is so rich with *good things* that the only things left to cut away are things that are also good, that I also really like. There are no remaining "give points," or obvious things to cut out that are hollow or unrewarding. I feel as if a lot of self-care tip books and articles assume that you are doing a laundry list of unfulfilling, obligatory, inappropriate commitments that you can easily cut from your to-dos as "no longer serving" you. My life is full, completely full, and it is full of deep goodness. So much goodness that it is too much and I am being swept away by a tidal wave of quality options, some of which will have to be sacrificed in order to continue keep my soul fueled. *So sad,* we laugh, *Our lives are just so hard, we have too many good things to do.* However, sobering again, I tell her what I told our Red Tent about three years ago: *I have already cut out so many things that I feel like the only thing I have left to cut off are parts of myself.* We are silent for a moment then, thinking.

Our conversation reminds me of the book I am re-reading, *Something More* by Sarah Ban Breathnach, a fat book of inspiration about digging through the layers of one's life that I first bought from a discount bookstore nearly twenty years ago. Something in the title and contents tugged at my soul, even though my life and being were in very different places than they are now. She is describing the author Vita Sackville-West's despair during a time of great creative abundance and success and how she wrote to her best friend, Virginia Woolf, *If I, who am the most fortunate of women, can ask, "What is life for?" how can other people live at all?* Sarah goes on to say,

> *So here we are...a group of talented, eclectic, even brilliant women. But at the end of the day, when we're finally alone, we're peering down into the black hole in our hearts. Our insatiable, inexplicable longing probes the emptiness.*

I reflect though that when I am alone I feel rich and full, a living tapestry of delight and meaning.

Earlier in the book, Sarah observes that it is tiny choices, day in and day out, that shape your destiny and weave your soul together, just as much as massive life changes and big decisions. She quotes Leo Tolstoy as writing:

> *True life is lived when tiny choices are made... Tiny choices mean tiny changes. But it is only with infinitesimal change, changes so small no one else even realizes you're making them, that you have any hope for transformation.*

I am reading Sarah's *Simple Abundance* as well, day by day, for the first time in many years. In it, she quotes John Ruskin about being happy in one's work:

> *In order that people may be happy in their work, these three things are needed: They must be fit for it. They must not do too much of it. And they must have a sense of success in it.*

There is no perfect.
There is no right way.
There is no secret that you're missing out on.
There is no permanent figuring it out.
No cracking the code.
No solving the puzzle.
No wrestling of the unknown into submission.
No taming of the mystery.
There is you.
There is the life you are living.
There is the seed of desire in your heart.
The whisper of longing from your soul.
Listen and choose
and then listen again
and then
choose some more.
It is all that can be done.

The Dream of Persephone

I have been asking for a dream of Persephone for two months and last night I received it.

There is a portal to the Underworld in the ravine on the enchanted acres across the road and through it, I meet Persephone. She is not the gentle companion and guide of my earlier images of her, she is fully in her Queen of the Underworld aspect, wild black hair streaming behind her, in a gown of red and black, with a commanding presence that is fierce, beautiful, terrible, harsh, and wonderful. She is asking something of me, setting me to a task: I am supposed to bring something back to her or let something go. In the dream I think I may write it down and I return from the Underworld into the leafy green, knowing that I have a date with Persephone to keep here in the future. In the rest of the dream, I am preparing for the journey, collecting things I will need, discussing what will happen. She is waiting for me and I have tasks to fulfill.

I awaken sharply and suddenly early in the morning, sun bright through my window, small child sleeping on my arm. The sensations of this encounter with Persephone are vivid in my mind, as is a sense of urgency and promise about completing my tasks. I lie still and try to recall the details of the dream, but I begin to slip back in and out of sleep and they become fuzzier and more distant. When I actually get up, thirty minutes later, after having dozed in and out, still clearly remembering that image of the wild, glorious, powerful black-haired queen of the night, but losing the finer sensation of what I was supposed to do with this information or encounter.

In the waking world, I enter the woods still in a dreamlike sort of daze, waiting for something. The air is cool again, the green feels fresh, I feel still and calm, while also curious. My dreamworld encounter with Persephone has shaken me a bit, as she did not seem particularly kind or welcoming and I wonder how much of my goddess imagery and relationship is attached to kindness. I consider that I have kept myself limited to only the Maiden aspect of Persephone. Sometimes in myth she is called Kore, meaning "Maiden." Before her Underworld journey, Persephone as Kore is tender and uncertain, needing guidance. I haven't touched on her rage, her power, her force, as she blooms into Persephone, the Queen of the Underworld.

This Persephone lingers in my memory: demanding, insistent, powerful. I find myself thinking about these encounters, the progress and process of this book, and whether people will think that I think I'm "special" or that I'm trying to be special. *Why do I think I'm deserving of any magical insight or experience?*

*I **don't** think I'm special though,* I reflect, *I think I'm just **noticing**, paying attention, to what is already there.* I hear the sound of crows starting to rise from the valley, very distant at first, and then growing louder and closer. The mean voice within me observes critically, *If you just **decide** something is magical that is already there and then every time you see it, you think you are having a magical moment, of course you will see that magic everywhere, and have those moments all the time.*

Hmm, thinks the kind self within, *exactly right. This **is** what happens.*

The sound of the crows continues to rise as I think about specialness and magic. I keep waiting, looking, waiting, and one flies out of the woods and lands right in a tree about twenty feet away from me. It is close enough that I can see its throat move with its harsh cry. I feel utterly enchanted and actually laugh a little with both disbelief and appreciation, special and magic are indeed both right here in front of me, I just have to go outside and look for them. The crow leaves nearly as quickly as it arrives and then one more crow arcs over my head on its way into morning.

Wild Streams of Living Truth

I want to saturate myself in wild streams of living truth.

These words run through my mind as I open my eyes to daylight. I take my youngest child to the bathroom and stop on the way back to peek out the window, the sound of a red-winged blackbird rising surprisingly from right outside. We lie back down for a few minutes to snuggle and the sound of the hawk pierces the air. Fragments of poem twine through my brain, insistent, curling, longing:

> *There is courage to be found*
> *in both rising and sinking,*
> *love to be found in dark corners*
> *and open spaces,*
> *poems to be woven*
> *of shells and bone,*
> *hope to be twined*
> *around crumbling hearts,*
> *wings to be witnessed*
> *unfurling*
> *into*
> *beyond.*
> *We hold the quiet*
> *we hold the storm*
> *and we dance between them*
> *on the rippling*
> *edge*
> *of the world.*

There is a thin and tender line between wanting things to be different and knowing they can change, sitting with yourself in all your feelings and letting them unknot, discovering you've actually been all right all along, wherever you are. I don't want to hold myself back by going solely on an inward journey, sitting on a rock in the same place every day, when perhaps I could be making new discoveries in new magical places everywhere I roam. But for me, this year, the inward journey has felt like *enough,* and what was being called for. I have shifted some attitudes, some habits, some mental processes, and this feels like it is enough for being happy where I am, being nourished by my environment, being enchanted by my every day. *Is there something more, though? Am I playing small, staying confined, remaining cocooned instead of flying?* If all I have to go by is my inner barometer, my felt sensation of what is "good" or "bad," happy or not, healthy or not, then I have traveled across leagues in the last two months.

This is the transformation that happens in "real life," in the cracks and edges of holding a family and business together, in the slices of morning sunlight, on the wings of crows, through the flowers blooming uproariously on roadside and meadow, and in the tall majesty of a pine tree on a cloudy day at sunset. This is the transformation that happened when I committed to making a change, to rebuilding my soul from the inside out, to listening to my center, to consciously evaluating my choices, actions, and patterns of thought, and putting myself back together right where and how I am.

I open my hands and reach out to Persephone.

What is the next task? What do I need to do now?

What is my next step? How do I know what to do now?

I feel restless and needy, wondering if what I'm doing even makes any sense. Am I crazy?

Cool air caresses my palms and curls around me.

Be *patient.*

You'll *know it when you see it.*

We're *not done yet.*

You *made a promise.*

W*ait.*

When is it time, I wonder, *to stop shedding and start rebuilding, inviting in, the things that I need? When will I be finished with the cleansing and letting go and be ready to explore the terrain that feeds my fire again, that makes me feel alive, purposeful, and connected, instead of wrung out and weary?*

Mark and I have talked a lot about my tendency, still present despite this journey of untying the knots in my inner landscape this year, to overdeliver, overprepare, and overdo, making myself miserable by doing too much with something I used to love, but have now drained of all life and power, by creating too much work for myself in association with it. I've told my friends and students about my practice of checking in with my Tired Future Self (or my Wise Future Self, or even just my Future Self). I do so want to always "do it all," and yet, as Jennifer Louden reminds us, I also have a "human-sized life" to live.

On the way back, I decide to step into the tiny temple for a few minutes. I sit on the couch, looking out at the rectangular patch of green and sunlight through the open front door. I remember the many rituals I've held here, the many things I've written and shared from this room, and I reflect that what I want to do right now, really the only thing I want to do, is to *write*. And to have ample time and space to have experiences that I can then *write about*. I do not feel inspired to hold groups, host rituals, or teach right now; I want to live, experience, observe, and record what I learn. I think about the intense agitation and despair that I encounter in so many people online, I watch the sunlight play against the waving grasses in my yard, way "too tall" by urban standards, but a plethora of living beauty and interconnection.

> *I want to remind people that the hawk flies,*
> *the crows trace a path across a white moon*
> *the grasses bend their heads in the sunlight*
> *the roses bloom*
> *all by themselves.*

I listen to Danielle LaPorte speak on core desired feelings and she makes a point that I have continued to return to this year, that it isn't necessary, desirable, or appropriate to expect "happiness" all of the time:

Happiness and feeling good all of the time are not the best metric of spiritual progress, enlightenment or even being well. I don't believe that it's humanly possible to be in your preferred state of pleasure all of the time. This is because we have human limitations, because we learn through contrast, because life is painful, and mysterious, and beautiful, and messy, and divine.

Let us not be despairing. Let us not give up hope. Let us see what lives and breathes and ripples and soars and blooms right in front of our eyes.

The Letter

I decide to write a letter to the daughter of a friend who has just turned eighteen and is moving away for college. I have known this girl for more than ten years, watching her grow from a nearly silent, determined eight-year-old (the same age my own daughter is now) into a poised, determined young woman. She attends a local community college already, but is preparing to transfer to a college in a city several hours away. This is a big step, especially for someone who was home-schooled for most of her life. Her mother has told me that she is very focused on her schoolwork, on getting good grades, and on doing well, at the expense of other interests and activities. Her mother is a little worried about her and tells me she has told her daughter that she needs to lower her expectations for herself.

As I write to this girl, I tell her that when I was nineteen I had just finished my bachelor's degree and left my hometown to go to graduate school at the same large school she is now planning to attend. One of my favorite professors at my undergraduate university told me I would need to "lower my expectations" for myself at the larger school because it was a much bigger "pond" (in my own smallish town I was a "big fish in a small pond"). I tell my friend's daughter that this still ranks as one of the most hurtful things anyone has ever said to me — it undermined my own confidence and made me feel like the people I trusted most didn't believe in me. It did not make me "relax" and be "easier on myself." Instead, it felt like a betrayal — like I was being told to "play small," when I knew I was capable of so much more.

I go on to encourage her never to dim her shine or play small in order to make other people feel comfortable around her. I have long known that when you are a driven and determined person, it can make other people feel insecure about themselves and their own efforts in life. It makes *them* feel better to tell you to ease up and to approach things with less drive. Being ambitious and devoted to your field are *not* bad qualities. They are not things to override or to feel shamed in. When you feel something deep in your heart and you truly want to pour yourself into it, trust that drive and let it move through you. I tell her what I wish my professor had said to me: *You are capable of excelling and of accomplishing great work. Never apologize for that or let yourself feel inadequate because someone else thinks you should be less intense.* In my own life, doing a "good enough" job usually doesn't feel good enough, because I know I can be *excellent*. Do not let anyone tell you that you can't be excellent, because you can be.

For the record, I *did not* have to lower my expectations for myself in graduate school. I was the absolute top of my class. But I never forgot how it felt to have that professor I looked up to and who I trusted tell me that I shouldn't try so hard. I hate being called an overachiever, because what I actually am is passionate and *devoted* to my own work and path. I achieve, yes, because I believe in myself, because I know I have it in me, and because I have the courage to push myself past what I might think are my own limits or limits others may try to impose upon me. It is true that your worth is not determined by what you produce—*you are always worthy*—but if you feel motivated from within to produce high quality work, that is a worthy goal too.

I tell my friend's daughter what I wish I could have heard:

Achieve away, dear girl! Be excellent! Do your own very best work. Never apologize for yourself. Take chances. Make brave choices. Stretch yourself. Know you can do it. Push if you need to. Rest if you need to too—it probably did take me way too long to figure that one out!
Nothing grows into its full potential without first having to push its way through the soil and out into the sun.

I tell Mark about my letter, feeling tender and vulnerable and with tears prickling behind my eyes. I tell him it is somewhat ironic that one of the knots I've been unpicking this year is the confusing tangle that I have created in my own life between worth and achievement, how I've been trying to learn how to not be so hard on myself and now I am encouraging this girl to pursue her dreams in an atmosphere and pattern that I recognize in myself as one that had lasting repercussions for how I continue to approach and experience my life. At the same time, I still stand by what I wrote to her. The thing is, I tell him, *is that it has to come from you.* The drive, the wish, the work, the plan, needs to be internally driven. And the choice to step back, to change, to let go, also needs to be internally driven and recognized. It has to come from *you*, it cannot be dictated by another who has decided you are "too much."

> *What if there is more*
> *than enough time*
> *for your unbound dreams?*
> *What if there is also time*
> *to build a tabernacle*

for tears
and to weave strands
of the ordinary
into your own holy text?
What if there is way
to dance prayers into being,
limits into loving,
hope into forever?
What if there is a path
to be carved through
an endless landscape
of mystery
in the mystical terrain
right behind your eyes?

What if you are more than you know,
less lost than you fear,
and whole
in your center?

What's Wrong?

Last night at a birthday party I tell a friend who is asking about Red Tent plans that I feel "evented out" this year. I'm worn by holding the space, by creating the container, by feeling responsible for everyone's experiences and needs. I'm not sure how to balance this with my own skill at event-planning, community building, and ritual facilitation. I also note with small concern that my loss of interest this year in things that used to bring me great pleasure is a worrisome sign. I do feel as if I have been on a journey to retrieve my joy, but *what is it that is making me close down, shut off, and withdraw from areas in which I excel and have found great enjoyment in the past? Is it burnout, or something deeper and more complex?*

I still have not figured out or discerned the "why" behind a lot of my work, it is layered together in a complex weave of natural skill, training, love, enjoyment, mission, dedication, devotion, and service *and* of proving my own worth, value, or purpose, and in some way, about earning love. As I unpick the knots of my own identity, I discover that I don't have to *do for* others in order to be a good person.

This morning I wake feeling constricted and chafed, like my life has become too small for me and isn't fitting right.

I feel into the gap I am feeling that has been created in my persistent mode of "too much to do," and I feel restless. While I have driven one mile away from home to various birthday parties, have had friends and employees in my home, and have visited with people, I have not actually gone anywhere further away. The last time I drove to town was thirteen days ago. *Isn't this what I have been asking for though? To draw in and away?* My life suddenly feels small, shrunken and I wonder if this is the result of exactly what I claim to have been craving: time to strip everything away and see what is left. *What if, when the to-do list is finished or laid aside, there is actually nothing left?* I have definitely noticed that all of these many projects that I *think* I just don't have time for, never rise into priority even when I actually do have more time. Perhaps I never wanted to do them anyway and that was just a story I told myself...

I remember *witnessing without fixing.* Perhaps it is simply *okay* that today I feel small and closed in and a few days ago I felt expansive with enchantment and dazzled by daily beauty.

What if I just allow myself to feel what I feel, to just let it be?

A hummingbird surprises me by buzzing right next to my head, perhaps investigating the red lining of my shoes, which are behind me on the stones. Another task floats across my mind: *Stop being so mean to yourself.* As soon as I give permission to feel what I feel without "fixing the feeling," trying to argue with it, or trying to make it go away, the sensation relaxes and I become still. I relax all my edges, feeling momentarily dissolved into stone, unable to tell the difference between myself and a rock. I wonder briefly about the dualism of mind, the differentiation I've just experienced between the intellectual, analytical self, the feeling self, the wanting self, the knowing self. These are wrapped up together as *me.* For me, though, there is nothing inherently wrong with this perception of multiple "selves" conversing within one being. It does not mean that "I" don't exist. It means that, as Whitman would say, I "contain multitudes."

Mark and I walk briskly at sunset. The air is less humid today and we move more smoothly, breathing easily. The roadside is dotted with pink wild roses and orange bursts of sumac berries amidst the ever-present tapestry of greens. As we come up the hill, we see a crumpled yellow form in the middle of the road. It is one of the birds we admired yesterday, dead. It is whole and perfect looking, except for an oddly extended leg. We surmise it was probably clipped by a car. We pick it up with leaves and lay it in the wild roses and cover it with oak leaves.

We speak of motivation and inspiration as we walk. I am trying to explain to him my feelings on this day, almost like I am "bored," which is an unfamiliar feeling to me. I tell him that I'm worried that in easing up, letting go, and untying my own knots, I might also be losing my motivation, my enthusiasm, my inspiration. If I am shedding being concerned with what people think or of needing to be approved of, *does that perhaps mean that I'm going to give up doing my work?* I tell him I have felt mechanical today, like I'm going through the motions, rather than feeling inspired. Then, I recognize that this is a gift, a blessing: to feel uninspired is such a rarity to me, such an unfamiliar state that it registers as something "wrong." Being inspired nearly constantly is so familiar to me, that it is my default mode. How fortunate I am to live and move and breathe in an environment where I feel steeped in inspiration most of the time. I tell him I'm experimenting with just letting the feelings *be as they are,* accepting that today I've felt mechanical, instead of trying to fix or change it. *But,* I caution him, *if my motivation, my spark, my drive, my inspiration is what moves our family and our business, we had better attend to it and work to guard and nourish it.*

Restless

After a restless night, I wake to bright sun and a clear sky. The temperature is cool, a breeze stirs the leaves. I feel distracted and taut, scattered and needy. I bring myself to the sensation of cool grounding in my feet on the rock. Even though I am out early, I hear no crows.

I reach out to Persephone again:

Persephone, please walk with me.

I need to know the next steps. What next?

I feel a small sense of desperation.

What if I have exhausted the possibilities? What if I can't figure out what's next? What if my exploration has come to end and I don't know it?

A red-winged blackbird begins to trill from a tree in front of me.

No *clinging.* No *forcing.* Be *patient.* Wait.

I see two mourning doves in a tree above the wild pink roses, and find an empty brown snail shell on the path home. I'm on the right path and I feel heartened to see it, especially with how dull and uninspired I've felt recently. It's almost as if I'm being reminded to return to the basics, to drop back down into the heart of the magic of place, and the steady, everyday miracles that are right here.

I have come to notice that with more spaciousness there is mental space left behind to ruminate and muse in ways that are often relatively pointless. My mind moves from old stories about teaching, to childhood, to early parenting, revisiting old hurts or embarrassing moments. I watch the squirrels teetering across delicately extended branches and I suddenly realize that I miss feeling *alive with passion.* Driven, yes, perhaps overly hard on myself, but inspired in my daily living by an overarching passion, a sense of meaning and purpose, a drive to *do my work.* Now, as I've laid things aside, I am no longer so certain as to what my work actually is. I think of my writing and how I want to focus on my books. As if in response, the wind picks up suddenly and a crow calls at the horizon line. Heavy raindrops stored in broad green leaves patter with emphasis across my shoulders.

I remember how devoted I once was to childbirth and breastfeeding education, the countless hours I spent on the phone helping tender new mothers navigate unfamiliar and challenging terrain. How often they called in tears, but hung up laughing, feeling understood. I used to be good at that. I remember how devoted I was to teaching human services classes, how I coaxed passion and enthusiasm and interest out of some of the most unmotivated and unlikely people. *Where did that person go?* I've craved the opportunity to lay so much aside and I am discovering that I now miss the person I was when I was certain of meaning and dedicated to purpose. I feel hollowed out and uncertain. I think about writing a practical manual of goddess-centered spiritual practice — in fact, what I thought *this* book was going to be. It takes shape briefly in my mind: essays, ritual suggestions, thealogical musings and I realize I am creating space in my life and world for this writing to be my act of service, my contribution, my dedication and offering.

Again, the wind picks up and my shoulders receive a spattered blessing from last night's rain. I hear the hawk cry, distant at first, making an unseen circle across the 180 degrees in front of me. I am alert, watchful, and it wheels into view, wings wide, cry certain and proud. I smile then, quiet in the green shadows. You do often have to wait, I find, to receive the day's gift. If you go inside from the woods too soon, you are likely overlooking the lesson that is offered to patient eyes and patient ears.

I realize I'm looking forward to some more inspiration instead of more introspection, a break from questioning and an invitation to some experiencing. However, I also think I'm finally recognizing this dusty terrain, this lull, this sensation of "what next?" for what it is. It is an opportunity. If I rush to fill it with senseless activity or old patterns of trying to be worthy, the opportunity I now have to consciously rebuild and create will be lost, swept away under a torrent of old ways of relating to the world, as well as the needs of others for my time, my life force, and my fuel. The fuel I have been so carefully gathering in and stoking deep within, so that I can feel it burn once more with passion and purpose, rather than as an energy source to be fed upon and depleted. A lull, a stop in a fallow field, the stagnant part of the pool, this is actually exactly what I need and what I've been steadily working on creating. I need it so I can consciously and mindfully choose my own *what next*, my own *why bother*, my own *why and how*. I need an unfilled expanse in which to explore, before I can build.

Our lumber delivery arrives on a big truck for the building of our work studio. The delivery person can't put it inside the building, so he unloads it in stacks outside the door of the greenhouse we are converting into our workspace. The sky is darkening with gathering clouds and there is distant thunder rumbling on the horizon. So we all get gloves, and Mark, our oldest son Lann, and I, move the heavy sheets of plywood flooring, piece by piece through the narrow door. We work in pairs, Lann and I trading off, Mark almost always being the one to have one end on his own. We are flushed and sweaty, arms dappled with small splinters, breathing heavily as the rain begins to delicately patter across the boards. As I move back and forth, I think about how my spiritual connection feels most present and real in solitude and stillness, outside of the mundane tasks of living: the movement of foot in front of foot, rough wood balanced against my shoulder, gloved hand slipping. So much of life is movement, not stillness. *How do we observe and move all in one?*

The Tenth Task

My head is aching. I have many things I could do, but I opt to step out of the family for a few moments, shutting the door to the bedroom for some silence and lie flat on my back on the floor. I drift and float for a few moments, feeling the muscles of my shoulders and neck loosening, my legs and arms becoming heavy and still. I become curious to notice that the sensation of having clothing on my legs has dissolved and it is as if I can no longer feel the presence of my legs, like my physical form has become diffuse and my edges have blended into the air around me. I wait within this sensation of dissolution for a while, noticing how it feels to not know where my body begins or ends, feeling dissolved, but not in a frightening way, in a soothing, peaceful, powerful way.

I think I drift off into some kind of sleep, but as I return to full awareness, it is with a clear thought ringing in my head:

Do not give up. This is it. This is the moment. This is what you've been waiting for.

I lie still, eyes open, a sensation of clarity descending. This is a moment of reckoning. This is what Persephone has been waiting for, guiding me to. I am at a crossroads now, one in which I can continue to do the work, to learn the lessons, to experience, to write, to move through this journey, this process, that continues to be revealed to me. Or, I can lay aside the "experiment" and pick right back up with my old habits, my old processes, my old ways of being and working. *Do I stay with it, even when it involves heavy rough lumber against my shoulder, and dead yellow birds in the road? Am I serious about what I've said I want to do, learn and experience? Do I truly want this work to move through me? Can I allow it? And can I allow the restless, acrid, painful, disappointing, or despairing pieces to exist and still keep going?*

> *The tenth task is:*
> *do not give up.*

I choose my cards of the day and receive the Pendulum card from Woman-runes. This is the rune of patterns: old patterns and karma. I smile in shocked recognition to see it, because this is exactly the gate of initiation I have passed through, the crossroads upon which I've made my decision, the pattern that was illuminated right before my eyes. To stay, go backwards, or to keep moving. I then remember something I haven't thought of since January: the Pendulum, in numerology, is actually my rune of the year for this year.

I am astounded by how much there is to pay attention to. How so many threads and connections weave themselves together with a mystical sort of patterned synchronicity that would have remained invisible without one step, one memory, one connection, or the fact that this year, I'm writing everything down and consciously bearing witness to the patterns as they unfold around me.

I discover that my headache has also eased, my mind is clear and alert and the inspiration I usually feel is flowing back down into my spirit. I reflect that there is a connection, obvious perhaps, between having a headache and my own sensation of withered connection, purpose, interest, and enthusiasm. When I am in pain, I feel dull and disconnected, as if I am going through the motions or forcing myself to respond or attend to the magic of the moment, the tasks I'd thought I wanted to do, the inspiration I had been following. When my head clears and my senses are restored to wholeness, I feel the channel of inspiration once more, the sense of purpose, the clarity of vision. These are physical realities and I need to remember to be conscious of how my perspective, outlook, and even sense of purpose or connection are shaped by pain or painlessness. It is certainly easier to feel like I live in a magical world when my head is clear and I feel buoyant.

I've been hard on myself, worrying that my "mood swings" and dips into despairing thinking and loss of interest in things I once enjoyed, swinging into energetic enthusiasm and excitement and waves of new inspiration, are signs of depression or perhaps even a type of cyclothymia. *Could it simply be that my emotional state is shaped by my physical experience and that physical brain pain, contributes to a sense of mental pain or disillusionment and confusion?* This seems so obvious that I feel silly, knowing how often I have said aloud as a headache eases or fades: *I feel my spirit coming back to me.* That is how I feel, restored to wholeness, completeness, satisfaction, soundness of mind, body, and spirit.

Thirteen

Today, my second son is thirteen and I now have two teenage boys. So far, having teenage boys is easy and pleasant. I expected more changes or upheaval, but instead they are still *them*. The most difficult thing about parenting them now is about how they get along, or don't, with the two younger children. The age gap between our children puts us into the position of needing to parent big kids and little kids at the same time, and the needs of the two differing groups are often at distinct odds. Last night this son, now teenager, asked me: *Mom, what is the dumbest thing you've ever done?* He pauses a beat and then adds with a laugh, *Have kids?*

I know he is joking, but I am serious when I reply that having him, specifically him—our second child—was the best decision of my life. I tell him that he transformed our experience of parenting for the better, that he brought joy into our family, that he changed the terrain of what it meant to have children, that he changed the landscape of parenting for us in the best possible way. He brought a priceless brotherhood dynamic in our family unit and that he taught us how meaningful, rewarding, and fun it can be to have kids.

He was born in a whirlwind labor, zooming into my life with dynamic passion, intense emotion, and heart with a force and power that has never ebbed. He was born when I surrendered my body to the freight train of labor and turned myself over to the might of creation moving through me. He was born in a bloody tangle of life and power that streaked my face, my arms, my legs, my chest, and even the bottoms of my feet with my own red blood and left a round, rusty stain on the concrete floor of our small cottage. His birth drove me to my knees and as the midwife passed him to me and I turned from my hands and knees into a sitting position and clasped him to my bloodstained chest, my older son cried out, *I like him, I like him!* We all still do.

When it was time to cut his cord, Lann stepped up to do it. And, as I nursed Zander in infancy, Lann would stand by my shoulder saying, *Zander, you have to drink nursies, so you can grow bigger and then you can play with me!* Zander has always been stalwart and loyal, firmly on the same team as his brother, ready to be friends from the moment of birth. Now, his voice is changing, hoarse and husky, because somehow he will be a man. He is only about three inches shorter than me, this person who once weighed nine pounds and slept with his head against my heart.

We open presents and I make him a pancake buffet with Nutella and fresh raspberries and whipped cream. I'm trying to figure it out, but I'm not sure how it is that we keep growing and changing and becoming new, and yet the same, people.

Belonging

I wake to bright sunlight streaming in the window from a whirling tangle of un-remembered dreams. I know there were places, events, people, lessons, and they all slip away from me as the new day dawns, leaving only tantalizing whispers of what I could have learned. There was something waiting for me there, in the dreamworld, I know, but it trails off into the morning, forgotten.

I step out into the cool air and bright sun. I hear the watery plinking of a blackbird and the cawing of a crow, very nearby: harsh, persistent, present. Instead of immediately going to the woods, I feel moved to check the mulberries, their broad, heart-shaped leaves hanging over the porch rail. I'm surprised to discover one red-black berry amongst the green and I eat what I find, savoring the pop and the delicate crunch of the many seeds, easy to eat, not sticking in your teeth in the manner of other wild berries. I feel delighted again, enchanted. The ennui from yesterday feels remote, as I tip my face to the sunlit morning, listening to the crows.

In the woods, I sit on the stones, watching the play of light and shadows, small in my green cocoon, the sounds of mourning doves rising up around me and my crow companion continuing to call to my left. I feel alert and engaged again, fully present, senses heightened, expectant and anticipatory, but unconditionally so.

I am paying attention. I am here.

A wind stirs through the trees, heavy with last night's rain and spatters the collected drops around me, but not a single drop touches me.

I am thinking of how people want to make a case for hopelessness, like the world is doomed. I am thinking about philosophers who want to make a case for meaninglessness. I feel like my purpose in life is to make the case that…

> *The world is alive with meaning.*
> *I can hear it in a thousand heartbeats.*
> *I can see it on a thousand wings.*
> *I can touch it in a thousand leaves*
> *I can taste it in a single, wild mulberry*
> *hanging red-black in the sun-striped green shadows.*
> *It is sweet.*

As I finish reading the book *Morning Altars* by Day Schildkret, I think about spiritual practices and rituals, thinking about how words and concepts drawn from Eastern traditions do not resonate or hold truth for me. They belong to other lands, other places, other times. My spirituality is rooted here: to *this land,* this place, this reality. I learned my magic and my rituals from being *here,* in this place, not from any externally imposed system. I do not feel the need for ancient texts to justify my prayers of being, my poems of living. I do not feel the need to study old philosophies or reconstruct old rituals in order to legitimize my path right now. My spirituality, my thealogy, my magic was born from this very ground.

I want to share the steeping
and the deepening,
the ripening and the blooming
of what it means to live,
not what it means to do it right.
I study surprise,
delight,
and unbound magic,
the dance of sunbeams with shadows,
the patterns of pine needles on
gray stone,
the spirals of seedlings
and seashells,
the prayers of waking and walking,
the anatomy of ensouled living
as it bleeds onto the page,
what quickens the heart,
what quiets the soul,
what catches the breath,
what delights the eyes,
what brings me home
into wholeness
and sets me down into my belly
full of awe.

The Hawk Cries (She is Here)

In my dream, nine geese swim on a lake that freezes, trapping one foot each and holding them there. My mind is whirling when I awake, trying to remember things, adding tasks that don't need to be worried about yet onto my mental list and then forgetting them, so that forgetting then becomes another thing to remember.

Everything is a part of the story, even the parts I don't understand yet.

I awaken to the sound of the hawk outside the window, high and distant. The air is cool and fresh, blessedly "thin" compared to last week's humidity. I feel so grateful to it, for being able to move easily. The stones are cool beneath me as I step onto them.

I think about my tenth task: *Don't give up.* This applies to so many things: don't give up and surrender to despair and hopelessness; don't give up and add everything chaotic and overwhelming back into your life; don't give up and neglect your morning practices; don't give up on your work, your promises, your devotion, your path.

Persephone, please walk with me.

I *am*. I *have been*.

Thank you.

There is a crashing flutter of wings near me, the sound of something rising up from the underbrush, but try as I might, peering through sunlight and shadow, I see nothing.

It occurs to me that maybe I'm still getting started with Persephone and that while the element I work with her on might shift, maybe she is the goddess of this whole journey of mine for the entire year. I think of my Underworld dream, her commanding, authoritative presence. Perhaps I need to consider shifting my relationship with her, my perception and perspective of her, rather than changing to work with another goddess too soon.

I have moved through an Underworld of my own making, but I still have much to learn from Persephone as Queen. *What am I forgetting?* I need to step from force and into choice. I have evaluated the beliefs and habits that are chafing at my spirit, but I have not yet risen into my self-sovereignty and become an active architect of my own realm. I have not discovered myself as responsible for my own choices and reactions, instead of feeling forced into responses by environment or obligation. I lift my hands in morning prayer and then go back inside the house, still musing.

In the workroom, I hear the hawk outside. I go out to look for it, but can't spot it. Its call dies away soon after I step outside and I honestly think it probably sees me without me seeing it and changes course.

An hour or so later, the hawk cries again. I go out immediately, squinting into the cloud-scattered blue sky. I see it this time, much higher than I would have expected for how loud it sounds. I've noticed before, in hawk watching, that sometimes you have to adjust your vision to look at the next layer "beyond" where your eyes would naturally focus and then *that* is where you see. I can see the sun glinting through the lighter color of its wing tips as it dips and soars and calls.

As I squint and stare, it begins to drop in circles, finally moving into a sort of dive that takes it over our roof and out of sight. Inside, my left eye has a lingering white spot from staring too close to the sunlight. I think it might be shaped like a hawk.

SUMMER

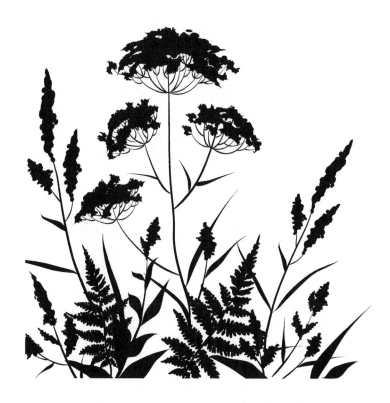

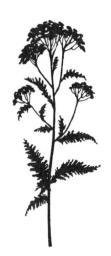

JUNE

Wild Strawberries

I am up early to go to the city for an annual Pagan Picnic event. The air is cool and peaceful. A cow is lowing insistently on the horizon line. The crows appear to still be asleep and the mourning doves also.

My sister-in-law picks me up. As we drive down the gravel road headed for the highway two crows flap ahead of us in the road. Around the bend, three vultures rise from the roadway, where they are eating carrion and as we pull onto the interstate a hawk wheels above the road, wingtips glinting white against the sun.

They ask me what I am writing about and it feels too vulnerable to say, so I make a joke that I'm worried I'm just keeping a list of all the crows I've seen this year.

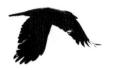 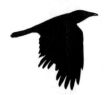

The Pagan Picnic is large and energetically overwhelming. I attend a presentation by a musician I enjoy online, but it is hard to hear her speak and sing over the exuberant chiming of an insistent gong being played by the woman teaching yoga in the next tent over. I recognize a familiar sense of disorientation and anxiety provoked by going somewhere unfamiliar—I always feel like I'm making the wrong choice or missing something somehow when I'm in a new place—I prefer going places the second time!

We walk to a distant bathroom with running water and I spot something red in the grass. I stoop to examine it and discover there are acres of wild strawberries right beneath our feet in this sprawling city park. Throughout the day, I spot them everywhere: beneath the blanket we spread to form a base to rest and talk, beneath our feet as we take a beginner's belly dancing workshop. I am charmed by the berries. They are my favorite part of this whole day by far.

I belly dance in the workshop with an old friend who has met us at the picnic. She walked with me through the tumultuous years of early motherhood, and we formed a bastion of support for one another as we traveled through uncertain landscapes and navigated the building of families. We are similarly unskilled with rhythmic, physical movement and it is with so much delight that we both move awkwardly together, shaking our hips and snaking our arms around in a circle with a group of strangers.

In the afternoon, we gather in a too-tight circle with unfamiliar, sweaty people for the main ritual. The theme of the ritual is perhaps too intense for a group of people who don't necessarily know each other or have any context for the working, but I do my best to lend my voice and my hands. We are asked what shame or fear we've been holding on to, cupping it tenderly to our chests, to our centers for a time, before releasing it. Mine is of having "too much to do." I set it free and hold my hope, my writing, in its place, plucking a small amethyst out of Pandora's box to remember my hope and what I can give.

Before we leave, I tell my friends I want to go take pictures in the strawberries. One friend seems bemused by my enchantment, asking me if we don't have wild strawberries where we live. We do, of course, but it is the incongruity, the juxtaposition of the tiny and wild beneath the feet of the many, with which I have fallen in love. When I kneel to take my picture, the front camera is still on from an earlier friendship selfie, and I catch a photo of my own face: sweaty, but illuminated with an afternoon sun shining right over my shoulder, a small smile on my lips, and a look of tender joy in my eyes.

I am excited and happy upon my return, buoyed by friendship, strawberries, sunshine, and song.

Chaos and Solitude

I rise before the rest of the family and lie on my belly on the deck in the cool air, reaching for raspberries. By hanging myself in the air from my waist, I am able to reach the three ripe berries I have spotted without having to navigate the weeds from the land. I sit and eat them slowly, gazing out at the tree line. I remember the coyote I saw on the rocks last year, sitting in the cool breeze. It was this same time, as the berries become ripe.

I take off my shoes and step onto the stones. I hear a heavy rustling sound and a strange chirruping note that I think is a bird, but it sounds like it is flopping somewhere on the ground instead of in the air or on a tree. I step quietly from stone to stone, barefoot and stand looking out. As my eyes focus closer to me, instead of at the horizon, I see there is no bird, but instead baby raccoons, climbing up a tree trunk. There are only three of them, though I'm nearly certain I saw four when I first encountered them two weeks ago. The mother is on the ground at the base of a large, dead oak tree. She catches sight of me and raises up, alert, staring at me like a small bear. She moves into the tree, climbing swiftly up the trunk and calls to the babies who leave their tree and trundle over to join her. She continues to make a sort of crooning sound, still keeping an eye on me as the babies explore the trunk and cluster around her body. Finally, given her persistent eye contact, I realize she is likely growling at me, not crooning to the babies, so I move back to my usual stone and sit down, where I can still peer at them through the trees.

I hear the sound of crashing underbrush behind me and while it is loud for a cat, that is still who I expect to see as I turn around, but it is a coyote, loping through the trees, only about ten feet away from me. It passes quickly, ears up, tail down, and I am stunned to see it. It is almost unbelievable that I was just thinking of my coyote moment from last year a few minutes earlier, assuming it would likely be the only close encounter with a coyote I would ever have. These woods, this place, the small adventures, magical moments and surprising encounters are countless, and I am honored to live and breathe among them.

I hear the hawk begin to call again and I can still taste the wild raspberries on my tongue.

A red cardinal lands on the tree just above my head, singing quietly into morning.

I go in to tell my family of my adventure, marveling that there is so much possible in such a small patch of land, wondering aloud how much I would see and discover if I stayed out all day instead of just for an hour.

The house is noisy and particularly chaotic, full of oceans of needs and undone tasks. The headache that I expected begins to build, first with blurry vision, noise sensitivity and distorted cognitive capacity and then affecting my joy, my projects, and my very sense of purpose on this earth, as self-doubt, disillusionment, and dissatisfaction creep over my brain. I am frustrated by the chaos of the house, the nonstop clutter and disarray, and speak sharply to my kids about it. Each harsh, burdensome word feels like it lodges in my skull, making my brain throb, my irritation hot and loaded with shame and self-accusation.

I recognize it this time though, stopping myself from continuing to push, eating a high protein lunch, taking an ibuprofen instead of trying to tough it out. I shut the door to my bedroom and sit alone for a few minutes to type. I am not surprised by this headache, it is what I term an "energetic hangover" from all the sights, sounds, and emotions of yesterday's festival. I remember these words from May Sarton's *Journal of a Solitude:*

> *There is no doubt that solitude is a challenge and to maintain balance within it a precarious business. But I must not forget that, for me, being with people or even with one beloved person for any length of time without solitude is even worse. I lose my center. I feel dispersed, scattered, in pieces. I must have time alone in which to mull over any encounter, and to extract its juice, its essence, to understand what has really happened to me as a consequence of it.*

I Dream of Hawks

I dream of hawks flying by the horizon line, bright feathers dropping from them, shed to fall in a twisting pattern to the ground. We walk along looking for feathers. I find a wing feather, long and slender, and patterned body feathers, softer and puffier than the strong wing feather.

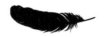

I wake early, but lie in bed for more than an hour, partially drifting in sleep, but partially reviewing my list of things to do and things undone. I am noticing how anxiety works in my body: it comes in a wave, with a hot sensation that settles across my upper chest and shoulders and prickles in a manner similar to embarrassment. It gathers in a knot behind my eyes, pressing, accusatory: *Don't forget, don't forget, do, do, do, and this. One more thing. You don't have enough time for everything. You can't do it all.*

This destroys joy. I feel these physical sensations so clearly, feel their sites of lodging in my body, that I worry about creating disease within myself. I have the sense that if I continue to let them lodge in these same places, digging fingers of insufficiency and pressure into my brain and heart, I may actually encourage illness to grow in those places.

The waves of hot anxiety continue throughout the day as I work. Eventually I confront the fact that there is no possible way to finish everything I have on my list. In fact, some of it I won't even get to touch. I feel parched and starved, chipping away at a ridiculously large mountain of my own making. I am at the verge of tears, again, when Mark gets home with the kids.

A friend who is taking my class writes to me and tells me that my level of inspiration is, "unprecedented among almost all human beings," and I let that soak in for a minute. Mark hugs me and tells me that he's never met anyone else with the capacity I have to create and yet still, I know, something has to give.

I am angry at myself for reaching this point yet again. I wanted to be through with this.

I tell Mark I wish I could figure out how to bring forth what there is within me, so much that wants to burst into life, to be communicated, taught, shared, written about, while correctly anticipating my own human limits and not boxing myself into a trap of my own making, where it becomes impossible to continue to perform and produce without unraveling from within. These things on my list, yet undone, are in reality things that only I have created the expectations for and then made the promise to produce and continue to fulfill at the same level of excellence month in and month out. I recognize that at some level I feel like creating products to sell, having a products-based business isn't as "worthy" as inspiring people, as teaching, or as coaching and guiding them. I feel like I need to do empowerment-based work because it is the "real work" and is somehow more "noble" than creating items to sell. The products-based work feels somehow less contributory: *what if I am just creating more "stuff" with which to fill people's lives? However, at the same time, what if it isn't about the worthiness of our products? What if it is that we, as a family, refuse to allow me the space and time to do that which I am called to do, am passionately driven to create? What if I feel like quitting because it is being crushed out of me, not because I truly want to quit?*

Mark kisses my forehead and tells me I'm amazing, and not to be so hard on myself. I feel a tiny bit like I'm being told to play small, to give up, to become less, to allow myself to become restricted and bound. I wrote about my sensation of burnout in the "Living the Questions" class I am teaching this year and got well-meaning comments and suggestions, but the cumulative effect is that I do not feel I have permission, anywhere in my life, to be vulnerable.

I'm on a Journey

The high, clear, musical chime of a distant bird greets me this morning, four notes in lyrical song: *dee-do-deeee-do*. It is a song I haven't heard since much earlier in the spring. I've never been able to glimpse the singer, but instead just enjoy its enjoyment of the morning.

In the woods, I take off my shoes. I still feel worn and defeated after yesterday's realizations and frustrated with myself for repeating the same patterns, but also, a type of anger at having the work I am doing driven out of me. It is hard for me to identify whether I want to withdraw from doing something because my own tendency to over-perform has destroyed it for me, or because the environment I've created around myself isn't one that supports the work I'm trying to do.

There are two crows conversing back and forth across the field this morning as I go out into the front yard to admire the first pink lily of the year, bobbing on a tall stalk laden with many buds. I stand under the mulberry tree, light filtering through the green, and listen to the crows as I pick a few ripe berries and eat each one. I walk over to look for the crows, but the conversation silences instantly, before I see anyone.

I feel peaceful and still, gazing out into a wall of green foliage.

I am on a journey, I think.

And it is true. I haven't been anywhere specifically, but I have been on a journey nevertheless, much of it invisible.

I am on a journey, and everything I think, feel, experience, witness, learn, do, dream, and notice is a part of this journey.

There is something whole and satisfying about this thought. Integrated. Woven together. Restored to self and being. Writing this book has contextualized my life and experiences in a satisfying way. I feel like the patterns of my own living have been made clear, brought to the fore, that my experiences, ideas, and capacities are weaving together into a complex, visible whole, that I understand myself in a new and deeper way, because I've been willing to learn *from myself* and to travel *with myself* into something unknown that is actually right in front of me and is right there within me. I feel more conscious, more intentional, more aware, and more present in how and *why* I am living, moving, creating, and being this year than any other, because I am consciously bearing witness to *everything that unfolds* and learning from what I see.

I hear the rhythmic rattle of a woodpecker begin and spot it at the very top of a slender, straight dead oak tree. It is small, black and white with a distinctive white patch on its back and a bit of red on its head. It rat-a-tats for a moment, tucks its beak into its wing and then repeats the process. I'm grateful to it for pulling me out of my slump, for reminding me that I *can* do my work, if I am clear and focused on what that work actually is.

The wind picks up, sweeping over my face like a cleansing breath, carrying away the tension and repetitive thoughts. "Not having enough time" is the next belief I need to release, I know it. At the same time, it feels uncomfortably true. I literally do not have enough time for everything that needs my attention, everything I want to do, everyone that wants or needs something from me. I am not sure how to restructure or re-approach something that does actually have a finite limit. Or perhaps it is just that I need to, *finally,* learn how to work with the actual limits of my days, instead of expecting superhuman production and capacity from myself day in and day out.

I wonder if I can ever embrace the fact that there is no "now I'll feel exactly wonderful all the time" point in my life. But that these daily dips and valleys *are,* in fact, part and parcel of a life lived mindfully, with intention and deep, vital engagement. "Yes, this too," Jennifer Louden would say. *Can I greet my life, and all of her experiences and emotions, with tender welcome?*

Yes, this too.

I set out to re-collect myself
to rebuild my spirit
and to reweave my dreams.
I moved through an Underworld
of my own making
and a canyon
of my own confusion
up a ladder of self-doubt
and despair.
One foot in front of the other
I continued
until upon a slab
of lichen covered stone
I took a deep breath
and discovered
the breath
the heart
the stone
were all made of mystery,
magic, and wonder
stirred together
in the cauldron of being.
Unknowing
may remain the only answer
and yet still we whisper
one more promise
to the wind.

It's Okay to Pause

Sometimes we have to say goodbye in order for our own hearts to continue to beat, I think. So we can hear our soulsongs again, so we can let ribbons of wonder trail through our days and strains of magic wind through our lives. So that we can have margins and space and softness. So we can remember what is really import- ant and know that we must care most about our own lives. No one else will do this work of caring *for* us, for it is our own task to tenderly care for who we are.

> *It is okay to pause,*
> *breathe,*
> *and be*
> *while the world*
> *keeps turning*
> *beneath your feet.*

I feel lighter and happier than I've felt in weeks.

I am making my goddess collage for the month. The last thing I do is choose which parts of a poem from the last month to apply, cutting the words out and often rearranging them into a new or composite form. Today, I collapse two sections of my "Cliffs of Questioning" poem into statements without question:

> *There is more than enough time,*
> *to weave strands of the ordinary*
> *into your own holy text.*
> *You are more than you know*
> *less lost than you feel*
> *and whole in your center.*

As I arrange the letters to fit my goddess shape, I find myself singing the words and discover they have become a song. I sing them high, soft, and sweet, and let them soak into me as I glue my words to the images of a mountain stream, soft moss, a butterfly, an open palm with a lotus across it, a dancing woman, and a watchful crow.

I draw a mandala on the final page of my art journal, begun so unexpectedly as a part of my writing class at homeschool co-op and then becoming such a treasured book of my own liberation. I use my rubber letter stamps around the edges to spell out:

You are whole in the center. Keep listening.

It is only noon when I finish all these things and I feel gleeful and excited, alert and happy, like I've shed something, again. Like I've been in a foggy place of wondering and I've felt my way back to the surface. I go out to water the plants and am surprised by a delightfully big box turtle moving slowly along the front porch, the orange spots on its legs brilliant and beautiful. The butterflies are dancing over the back deck, orange wings opening and closing in the sun.

We go to the river for this week's family potluck, wading in the spring creek, and eating taco salad and sharing stories. It is the first time in about six weeks when it is just us, my parents, two of my siblings, my sister-in-law, my kids and their two cousins, instead of hosting some kind of event or party or having an "occasion" to be together. As I stand alone in the icy cold spring water of the creek, watching white and black dragonflies land on rocks and green and black dragonflies dance around them, I remember a poem-musing from last year in which I asked:

> *What if you were to sit*
> *by the river of your own life*
> *observing the current*
> *watching the flow,*
> *sensing the depth,*
> *feeling the rhythm,*
> *and not needing*
> *to tell about it,*
> *but instead taking*
> *a long, replenishing*
> *drink?*

I think the moment in which I wrote these words actually was the start of the slow process that has been building in me ever since.

The Fall

I dream of a monarch butterfly, emerging from a chrysalis and spreading broad orange and black wings out across the leaves. It is surrounded by a sort of white foam and is drying it out in the sunshine.

I think about all the sorrow in the world, all the fear about climate change and human violence, and I remember the wild foxgloves blooming white across an abandoned meadow. There is a part of me that feels like there are certain people who want us to stay trapped in fear and overlook the foxglove. In this moment, I feel like I am here to tell people that it blooms and blankets the meadow with beauty.

It has been three months since I started writing every day. I think about this new passage or transition I have been through. It takes time and devotion and courage to actually, genuinely *change* one's own habits of thought and patterns of relating to oneself. This is about really *living through and into* what I'm learning, not just writing about it and wrapping it up into a tidy conclusion. This is messy. It is complex. Really *changing* takes time, attention, and devotion.

Some days I feel frustrated with myself like I simply can't learn anything, like nothing I am discovering has stuck. Some days I feel like I've traversed impossible terrain and reached surprising depths and heights, just from my own small corner of the world. Through each of these feelings, I continue to trust the book. To trust the story. When I reached my personal limit with an untended spirit and truly determined it was time to rebuild my soul, I set out to do it using the materials available to me in my own back yard: trees, stones, birds, sunlight, moss, and morning. I feel grateful to myself for having the courage to do it, to not wait for "later," to not assume that I need to make a physical pilgrimage to another landscape, to not form a more complex or demanding series of conditions for myself before I can begin, but to just do it and to keep doing it and keep doing it, through every glittering moment and every rocky shadow.

I take my daughter to Girl Scouts. On the way home, thin, smoky fingers of lingering twilight streak the sky like we are peering behind a veil into an alternate reality. We see a dead deer, a dead raccoon, a dead fox, and a dead snake on the road, each a pang to us, a life that didn't have to end. Shortly before turning into the driveway, we see red eyes in the road, we get closer and see it is a bird, sitting in the road. It looks hurt, but as we pull alongside it, it suddenly disappears. A few feet beyond our car, we see red eyes in the road again. We creep up and it is the same bird. *It must be hurt,* we say. But in that moment it takes off and flies away into the woods. We think it might be a whippoorwill.

I am so ready to be home, eager to get inside, reviewing my remaining plans for the day and thinking about my day off tomorrow. The kids dawdle slowly in front of me, I ask them to walk a little more quickly, but they don't, saying, *Mom, we're already home!*

As I step up behind my daughter who is opening the front door, my right foot slips down the step and I fall, hard, my ankle twisting beneath me in what feels like a 90-degree angle inward, like I have stepped down onto the end of my leg instead of my foot. I have dropped all my books and bags as I fall and am left crumpled in an awkward sitting position, my leg hurting in a different and deeper way than I've ever experienced before. Mark comes running and I say, *I think I've really, really hurt myself.*

I have to crawl indoors, my ankle feels tender and puffy and you can see the swelling already, even through my sock. I can't move my leg and so I sit in the recliner with it awkwardly twisted against the footrest. My first thought is that I have broken it and that I can't have broken it because I need to work. *How will I work?*

I feel strange and depersonalized, like I'm separated from myself, talking fast and repetitively, analyzing my own trauma and my own responses and experiences as I speak. I don't cry at first, but then when I start to ramble about how I won't be able to go on a walk with Mark, won't be able to go to the woods, my face crumples and I cry and cry, interspersing my tears with gales of hysterical laughter about how silly I am, how I wasn't *doing anything,* I just, weirdly, inexplicably, pointlessly, fell down. My kids watch me helplessly. I review the details several times, learning nothing new. We look at the puffiness, it feels weird, like my ankle is encased in something. Pain throbs up into my shin over and over again. I move my toes a little. I feel like it might be broken, like we need to go to the emergency room.

I decide to stop calling myself dumb and make a reiki symbol on my palm and lean down to give myself reiki. As I do, I feel the pain subsiding, the puffy sensation easing. I ask for arnica to take. I ask the Goddess for healing, for strength, I pour her love into my ankle. I tell my swollen and bruised flesh and bones that they are good and strong and we're going to be okay. Behind my closed eyes, a heron flies across gray-streaked sky.

My leg no longer throbs and I feel calmer, more trusting. I have a strong sense that I'm going to be okay. I crawl to the bathroom to get ready for bed and then hop on one leg to the bed, propping it up on a cushion, with an ice pack.

A Sign?

I dream of the hawk diving through blue sky.
I dream I am walking and my ankle, though tender, is okay.

I wake to the sound of rain and birdsong and my leg still elevated on the pillow exactly as it was when I fell asleep. I slept well.

But as soon as I start to move my ankle hurts, and I know I am not magically all better. This will take time. As someone whose life has been shaped by wings and walks this year, this is a hard circumstance to swallow. I feel like an invalid and I hate it. Usually I move swiftly through my days: capable and certain. It is strange to have gone from fully mobile and strong, to tender and vulnerable, in the space of one step.

Of course, I wonder if this is a "sign," an enforced mandate to slow down and to rest. But then I remember a promise I made to myself two years ago when I developed a nasty sinus infection after caring for my sick kids: if I would never look my sick toddler in the eye and asked him what he had done to "deserve" being so sick, I would never visit that cruelty and needless blame-casting upon myself.

Mark makes me tea and I listen to the birds and the rain. I lie with my ankle propped up and work on my outline for our Red Tent retreat this coming weekend. I hear the hawk begin to call and long to be outside looking for it. It is amazing, and cliché, to realize how much I take things for granted, and how I just blithely assumed I'd continue visiting the woods and walking two miles on the road with Mark every day this year.

I feel shaky and kind of sick when I get up and hop about, trying to take care of a few things that need my time and attention. I retreat back to my bed and read to my kids for hours, drinking chamomile tea, choosing my cards for the day, thinking, and placing supply orders for the shop. I don't feel motivated to journal or write or draw or listen to podcasts. I feel dull and constrained, anxious and unknowing, confused and incapable.

My mom comes to bring me crutches and arnica gel and I tell her that I feel like I have *one day of this* in me and that's it. Then, I cry. I know that there is so much further to go.

Thunder rumbles through my open window, the mulberry tree is heavy and green. I can't see anything else. I think about the yarrow tincture I was planning to make. The rain begins.

After dinner, I sit in the recliner growing increasingly irritated with my family, all these able-bodied people walking around and not taking care of anything that needs to be taken care of, just waiting for orders to be barked tiresomely at them from the chair. Finally, I cry and say I need to get out of here, even just for a few minutes. I hop and then crawl to the back door and lower myself out onto the rain-wet deck. Tiny bits of pink and blue still cast puffs of light across the darkening sky. I look with longing at the path to the woods.

Tanner comes in and out, checking on me, telling me to scream for him if I need help getting back inside. I cry some more, sitting in my little crumpled pile, and a whippoorwill begins to call in the night. I reach out with my Persephone prayersong.

> *Persephone,*
> *please walk with me.*
> *May I pace myself*
> *with grace.*
> *May I honor my limits.*
> *May I trust my body.*
> *May I celebrate my enthusiasm.*
> *May I be patient*
> *with the constraints*
> *of time*
> *and this small human self*
> *in need of care.*

I Dream Everything is Okay

I dream I am walking and everything is okay.

I wake to sunlight and cool breeze and the low, quiet sounds of a mourning dove calling into morning. I have slept well. My ankle feels fine from here, like I'd hardly know anything was wrong, but when I get up, I can't walk on it. I feel small and caved in, like my world has shrunk into nothingness, with just one little unforeseen change.

I feel irritated with myself for not being more resilient or courageous or even cheerful in the face of a relatively small injury. I feel whiny and plaintive and wish I was stronger in my attitude. I think about all the people who cope with chronic pain and serious injuries that impair their mobility every day and feel bratty and spoiled. I then grant myself a small amount of grace — this was very unexpected and I've only had a few hours to adapt, to adjust my expectations, to bolster my resilience, to develop coping skills. I do not need to add self-criticism to my list, I simply need to work with what I have and discover what I can. But I am so frustrated. It is difficult to be brought to my knees, literally, by a small change in physical health. It is disappointing to become so easily despairing and hopeless. It is disappointing to not be able to rally myself with my usual strategies or be alert for the new gifts within this unexpected, forced reprieve (I *did* say I was trying to figure out the difference between choice and force!) and instead just slip into a kind of shadowed apathy, where everything feels too hard to even try. I am frustrated that I can't magically embrace an enforced mini retreat, rest and restoration opportunity.

I have been musing about the difference between choice and force and this physical limitation highlights for me what it feels like to have an externally imposed limit instead of a self-imposed limit. I think about all the yoga poses you can do without standing and guide myself gently through a slow series of lying down, seated, and kneeling poses.

My leg begins to ache more and I notice I am pushing. I feel dizzy and a little sick, eyes blurry, body feeling battered. I go to lie down and sleep for two entire hours. When I wake, I am disoriented and think it is the next morning, think I need to prepare for the employees. When I realize it is evening and not morning, I feel grateful, like this is "bonus time."

I creep outside into the greening shadows and sit on the deck with mosquitoes flying around my head, feeling the air. It is instantly soothing and restorative to be outdoors, I feel my spirit coming back to me, I feel myself being renewed and replenished as I tilt my face to the waxing moon.

> *Persephone,*
> *please walk with me.*
> *May I balance creation*
> *with restoration.*
> *May I balance*
> *expression*
> *with contemplation.*
> *May I balance exuberance*
> *with stillness.*
> *May I balance giving*
> *with receiving.*
> *May I balance fire*
> *with flow*
> *and blazing*
> *with simmering.*
> *May I balance generativity*
> *with renewal.*
> *May it be so.*

The Eleventh Task

If this is a midterm exam, integrating the lessons that have come before, I may be failing. All my lessons of the year are brought screeching in, messages and tasks undone, unapplied. If there ever was a time to rest, take a break, allow margins, now is the time. If I have been musing about choice versus force, now I am experiencing actual force, limitation that is not self-imposed or mental, but physical, which seems to be reactivating old mental patterns as well.

Movement is magical and I miss it, I think, sitting on the deck this morning in the cool air, watching the mulberry leaves.

May I remember that watching and witnessing is one of my most precious and powerful gifts.

May I soften into limitation, relax my striving, ease my straining, and relax into resting.

A mockingbird flies onto the porch and lands briefly on the windchimes. An orange butterfly opens its wings gently as it rests on the outer wall of the house. The lilies are full and gorgeous in the sun and a new rose has opened.

I lie down on my back with my eyes closed and breathe.

> *Goddess of the sacred pause*
> *please grant me the courage*
> *to lay aside swiftness*
> *and take up slowness,*
> *to embrace limitations as learning,*
> *silence as stabilizing,*
> *waiting as worthy,*
> *and sitting as divine.*
> *Goddess of the sacred pause*
> *help me to know stillness as strength,*
> *patience as powerful,*
> *and healing time*
> *as holy necessity.*

I hear the hawk call begin, high, faint, and distant.

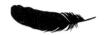

We catch up on shipping for many orders, our employee helping me to put goddesses into bins, get books out of boxes off the floor, and lift tubs off shelves. I am struck by how often I am usually up and down through the workday, flitting from here to there like a butterfly, now stationary, my wings hobbled into pointing and requesting instead of lifting and doing.

My mom brings back my little kids and we talk about our river retreat plans for the next day. She comments that I seem cheerful, less defeated and depressed. She's right. I don't want to be doing this, but I *am* working with it.

After the workday is officially complete, I go outside to breathe, tip my head to the remainder of the sun. I watch orange butterflies on each bloom of magenta milkweed dotted in the back yard. I lie on my back on the deck and look up at the sky. The clouds are still in a patchwork of blue. I close my eyes and let the breeze sweep over me, the ache in my back and ribs seeps away.

I remember…

The eleventh task is:
witness without fixing.

Red Tent at the River

I dream I am leading a summer ritual for families. I haven't prepared in advance and I'm weaving together elements spontaneously from my memories.

I awake to the sound of rainfall outside the window and the feeling of a soft gush of blood between my legs. It is nearly the June full moon, I've been spotting for a few days. Today is Red Tent at the river, it is all aligned. I feel momentarily full of inspiration and enthusiasm, hopping up—tenderly—and typing in the darkness with my notes for Red Tent, for the dream-inspired family ritual in July.

I step outside cautiously. The rain has slowed, the deck is slick and wet. The Queen Anne's Lace is bowed down, broad white flower heads almost touching the ground. Raindrops sit picturesquely on the roses. I lean on the railing, looking wistfully at the misty path.

I miss you, I say.

We miss you too, is the reply, *you belong here.*

I bake two cakes and make a double batch of homemade custard for a Father's Day trifle tomorrow. This uses up my slender thread of upright stamina, so I go back to bed, where I listen to my kids arguing and making assorted loud and pointless noises.

My mom comes to pick me up for our Red Tent retreat at the river. I am shocked by how unstable and unsteady I feel on the uneven terrain outside. I've been getting around fairly well indoors. Stumbling over countless rocks and dips of earth, I feel flung back into the original injury, barely capable of standing, let alone hoisting myself along. I put on the orthopedic boot she has from her own past ankle injury and while it feels cumbersome and as if it is throwing my other hip, knee, and ankle out of alignment, I no longer feel as if I'm about to damage myself further with one wrong step. I feel vulnerable and small, invalid, tender, not a complete person.

My friend and my mom work setting up the simple ritual site and I watch, seated on the pavilion's porch, marveling at their adept and fluid movements, their bodily capacities. The blankets are spread beneath swaying green trees on the point of land overlooking the confluence of two creeks and the river. We can hear the breeze and the gentle flow of the water. Women start to arrive, full of hugs and smiles and words of connection. I hobble to the blanket and sit down, where I can show my bruising. My chiropractor friend has traveled all the way from Kansas for our circle. She examines my ankle with care and a light touch, telling me it probably isn't fractured and though it may take six weeks, I will get better.

We gather in circle and I guide them briefly through a grounding. A light breeze rolls around us, caressing our faces and our closed eyes as we rest our hands on one another's lower backs and hum together, surrounded by green trees, under a wide blue and white sky. A chorus of bugs and birdsong joins with our voices, the gentle drift of the never-ending river current hums, the ground is warm and whole beneath our feet.

I have asked four of my friends to offer an elemental blessing with some herbs of the Summer Solstice. They circle us, speaking their carefully chosen words, scattering herbs to encircle our working. We sit and sing together, words of welcome and affirmation, love and wonder. Tears begin to fall from several women as the songs soak into our bones. I'm not sure what brings the tears: the circle, the song, the container, the sunshine on our shoulders... I look up to see four vultures cresting the bluffs and circling our circle with their own.

We are here, we are alive, we are whole, we are well.

We pass the rattle and I share my progress with soul rebuilding, how I've determined to write myself back into being and how I am succeeding in that. I speak about the impact that my injured ankle is having on my ability to shape and frame my experiences. I tell them that the book began with them, sitting in circle, witnessing my words, holding space for my promises and woes.

We break for snacks and conversation and begin our projects, stamping designs on muslin tarot bags and doing batik dyeing. First, I stand to talk with a troubled friend, but my left leg begins to ache as I lean awkwardly on it while the orthopedic boot encases my right leg. My mom drives me to the cabin to use the bathroom and I tell her I think I'm overdoing it, I feel frayed and weak. I know it is because I'm expending too much energy supporting the circle energetically, holding the space, the power, the safety of our container. She suggests I put my foot up and rest for a spell, and I do, letting the women bring me strawberries and crackers.

I feel recharged with food and more capable and we move to our next item, an experimental, body-based concept I'm not sure will fly with our group, as it feels very intimate and personal. We divide into groups of four and take turns lying down on the blanket in the center of our small circles. The women around us gently lift up parts of our bodies and lay hands upon us offering the wish, the hope, the blessing: *let go.* While we occasionally laugh and some part of us initially feels silly, we quickly relax into the power of what we are experiencing together. This sun, this wind, this grass, these trees, this river, it all bears witness to the care with which we treat one another. It is surprisingly personal and intimate to be handled so gently by our friends. I am surprised by the tender feelings I experience when being the recipient of touch and in giving touch to others. I place my hands on both sides of a friend's face and see the tears well up and spill over beneath her closed lashes.

We re-gather in our larger circle, feeling connected and supported in a new way, and sing together two songs of letting go. The rest of the women go to the river for a ritual immersion and cleansing after our letting go ceremony. I can't accompany them, so I wait on my blanket, singing another song: *Let it in, let it go, round and round we flow, weaving the web of women.*

I sing for a long time, high and quiet into the gentle air. A vulture turns lazily above the river.

A friend brings a cup of fresh spring water back for me and drizzles it slowly over my ankle, healing me with a bit of spring immersion too.

The Woods are Calling

Thunder crashes against the window and rolls along the sky. Rain falls heavy and wild. Tanner crawls into bed with me. Since I can't go outside, I linger in bed, small boy's head against my shoulder, breathing deeply. I notice that allowing time for this moment holds magic too: connection, security, peace. *You smell like love,* he tells me.

The gift in this setback has really been to recognize, as perspective often demonstrates, how much I have. I have spent any number of hours this year fretting over not getting to do something and feeling resentful of being impeded in my progress. Now I am actually unable to do something and actually imped-ed, and it throws into sharp relief the freedom and influence I have enjoyed the rest of the year — it is much clearer to me now how often I don't do something for a multitude of other reasons that are within my own control and choice, not because I "can't" or I am not being "allowed to."

The rain lifts before midday and orange butterflies begin to dance around the mulberry trees. After I finish a limited, gentle yoga practice, I hear the hawk begin to call, high and distant. I make my way slowly to the back door, thankful my mobility is increasing dramatically every day. I step out carefully into the humid, deep sunshine. A black and white dragonfly lands on the rosebush and green dragonflies dance over the wild berries. I am sad that I can't go off the deck to pick them. We listen to the hawk. It is very high and we can't spot it against the sun glare in the blue sky. I hear two crows talking back and forth to each other in the woods and it is irresistible. I must follow.

I tell my kids I'm going to try it and I set off for the woods, slow and teetering on the uneven ground. I am barefoot for increased perception and navigation, water seeping up through the moss under my feet. I feel weak and unsteady, unsure if this is a good idea, feeling perhaps I should turn back, because I never noticed how many rocks there were underfoot before that are angled in such challenging ways, not flat and navigable. What irreplaceable treasures my strong legs, ankles, and feet have been to me for forty years, carrying me across sand and stone and hill and valley, without fail. I creep on and finally emerge, duck-ing under the hickory tree and onto the flat stones, feeling such relief and peace sweep through me that I almost cry.

The rock is wet and I am careful to guard against slipping, moving onto one stone only and immediately sitting down. I watch the play of light and shadow across the blue, purple, and yellow bruising on my ankle. It is afternoon, but I notice the cedar tree by me is still glowing in the sun. There is undergrowth disturbance in front of me, but no matter how carefully I peer I cannot see what it is moving there, beyond my gaze.

I see a fallen branch propped against vines. With the way the sun is striking it, it looks like a snake with its mouth open. The breeze stirs around me. I look away from the snake stick and when I look back, I can't see it. For a moment, I think it must have been a real snake, but then I readjust my head and it appears again, striking motionless into the air.

I place my palms flat against the rain sodden stone. It is cool and solid and I let its strength soak into my hands. Then, I draw my leg into my chest and place my cooled hands against my ankle. *Stone strengthen me, reknit my bones.*

As I sit there, stone power soaking into my flesh, symbolically (or perhaps literally) remineralizing my body, I ask Persephone for healing.

> *Persephone,*
> *please walk with me,*
> *goddess of choice and surrender,*
> *goddess of change and renewal,*
> *goddess of determination and desire,*
> *goddess of loss and love.*
> *Underworld companion*
> *of luminous darkness*
> *and shadowy light,*
> *please guide my steps*
> *and inspire my courage,*
> *as I uncover my way.*

Too Much, Too Soon

My ankle feels extremely stiff and swollen, unable to bend, and I worry that I've pushed my luck with my ambitious movement.

I am surprised by how often I connect this injury experience to my recovery postpartum with each of my children, remembering supporting myself on the shower wall, blood dripping down my legs; rolling painfully out of bed, straining my bruised and torn tissues trying to hobble to the bathroom; lying alone in the bedroom not wanting to call, yet again, for help; feeling weak and needy and not wanting to need help or to micromanage the help needed. I begin to recognize that those postpartum experiences really have been, mercifully, my only other real experiences with feeling wounded, tender, vulnerable, and needy. The experience of going from strong, healthy, and capable to suddenly wounded, injured, and helpless, is one I've only experienced after giving birth. It always bothered me to feel so weak after having been such a strong, healthy, powerful, roaring, energetic birthing woman.

These postpartum experiences were Underworld journeys too, of descent and renewal, navigating my way through a new terrain of identity, shedding parts of myself and refashioning and rebuilding myself anew from the ragged scraps and bleeding edges. Pregnancy, labor, birth, and postpartum are a labyrinth that requires careful, slow, sometimes painful, navigation. There is a journey to collect your baby and to return with the child in your arms, bleeding, wounded, rising. I tell my childbirth class students that the labyrinth of birth and parenting is not a maze, you can find your way through it blindfolded, crawling if you need to, but somehow, eventually, you will find yourself blinking in the sunshine, carrying new life in your arms.

"I wish I could say what I really mean and be heard." I wrote these words when I was a tired and tender new mother less than three months postpartum, aching for who I used to be, struggling to integrate this new self, immersed in the forge fires of early motherhood, longing for the strong hand of love in mine and starving for myself. Sometimes I still feel this way. I wish I could express how I feel: thready and worn, ragged and alone, gasping and breathless, awash with anxiety and panting before the mountain, while also expressing how I am alive with purpose, blazing with ideas, burning with enthusiasm, flushed with passion. How I am sometimes stunned by my own brilliance and often humbled by my own weariness and the sensation I've created something too big for me to hold while simultaneously wanting to do even more.

I am here, now, in a new labyrinth of recovery, hobbling my way through the twists and turns, crawling when I need to, straining to peer around the bends, step-by-step, I am coming back home to myself.

Forcibly Grounded

I creep quietly outside while the rest of the house sleeps. I feel pudgy and forlorn, like my leg muscles are atrophying by the second. My head aches. I am uncertain of where I stand (when I can't stand) and unclear about my next steps (as they are difficult to take).

I feel adrift and uncertain. I'm not sure where to go from here, if I should switch goddesses, switch elements, hold a closing ceremony on the rapidly approaching Summer Solstice, or if I should keep working with Persephone and with Air. Maybe I need to switch my element to Earth, but not the goddess with whom I work. Maybe my walk with Persephone is longer than I knew it would be and it will not fit into a tidy box or a clear system. Every time I ask the question today, and there are many times as it is foremost on my mind as the Solstice approaches, I see a vulture through the waving trees.

When I return indoors, I try to talk to Mark about my journey and muse about what, if anything, I'm supposed to learn from this experience. I feel like my ankle injury, this unexpected setback, is unraveling the contextual elements of my own personal journey of the year and cutting me off from the inspiration and context I was relying on to frame my story as it unfolds. He suggests that maybe I have been forcibly "grounded" and it is time to work with Earth, now. I wonder if I have relied on the woods as a "crutch" (ha ha!) to fuel me for too long and I'm being challenged to stretch and grow, to find new spiritual resources, reserves, and communication, somewhere else, maybe even just inside my own home, maybe inside myself. Maybe the woods have been too easy, maybe I've come to rely on them too much and have not continued to develop, to stretch myself, to grow, to move fully into these processes and layers of unfolding.

I settle myself onto the ground, my thoughts return to the elements.

Earth is for stabilizing. Earth is for grounding. I have cast a lot away on the winds, I have let a lot of mental patterns unwind in the breeze. Maybe it is time for me to stabilize myself, bolster my reserves, build myself from the ground up, strengthening my foundation, my feet on this earth.

Persephone, please walk with me.

I *am.*

How do I know what to do next?

A lone vulture trails by on ragged wings.

I start my audio recording task and have only spoken for a few minutes when I finally spot the hawk that has been calling insistently, coasting low and brown through the trees. Before I can finish pulling myself awkwardly to my feet to step out to get a better look at it, it is gone, up and away, beyond my sight.

Thunder rolls and crashes as I speak into my recorder and then slender rays of light snake down between the gray clouds. A crow glides swiftly by, something carried in its beak. I make three different recordings. The hawk doesn't stop shrieking, though I never can see it, insistent and piercing, around and around the fields and trees.

I decide to go inside to finish my workday at the computer. As I type, update, schedule, and maintain, far away, high and clear, the hawk continues to call against the gray sky.

Who are you without your symbols
and your striving
when you are ragged in your skin?
Who are you when you are stripped bare
laid raw
unknowing and alone?
How do you know how to rise
when you have fallen,
fly when you are hobbled
and soar when you ache?
Where might you soak
in a deep pool of truth
until your bones knit back together
and you rise shivering into
a moonlit night
full of fire?
Can you scoop hope back into your arms
re-collect yourself from where you've fallen,
gather your tattered edges
and lay down new seams
with bright threads of possibility?
Can you shed your skin
cast off your longing
spread your wings

steep your meaning
into a strong,
sweet
concoction
of renewed truth,
purpose,
and vision?
Can you lay it all down
and then pick up what you still want
and re-weave your heart,
truth,
spirit
with lumps, bumps, passion, and power
all entwined?

Inanna's Descent

I wake thinking of snails, snails on green leaves, slow, slow, slow.

I lie on the deck under sky so solidly gray-white it is almost blinding. I have to squint up into it. The blackbirds sing. Mosquitoes twirl around my face and arms looking for a feast. I've placed my head near the roses and I can smell them as I endeavor to still myself, to sink into presence, to witness what is. New blackberry leaves are right by my face and I see small, delicate dewdrops clinging to them, a light silver frosting on the burgeoning green stems.

I once more feel cut off, adrift, this ebb and flow of life and sensation. If I thought I was in the Underworld before, I didn't realize the extent of the descent.

I wonder if Inanna would have been a better myth to guide my steps, because I feel like I'm starting to descend through another layer, stripped of my talismans and shaking in my skin.

I meet Inanna for the first time in firelit darkness. I am at a midwifery retreat in mid-Missouri, a baby at my breast, preparing to teach a workshop about birth art and celebrating pregnancy through art. The spellbinding and measured tones of the birth educator in front of us spins the tale of Inanna into the gathering night, before an audience of fundamentalist Christians and hippie pagans alike, as we sit around a flickering campfire. I am in love.

She tells of Inanna's Descent, her renewal, and return, an ancient Sumerian myth, inscribed on weathered clay tablets by the first named poet in the world (well, in recorded human history), Enheduanna, priestess of Inanna.

She shares how Inanna journeys through seven layers of descent, seven passages of initiation in order to confront her sister, the Queen of the Underworld, Ereshkigal. At each gate, she must lay down something of herself, something precious, something powerful, a symbol of her own identity, until she arrives in the Underworld naked and shaking, stripped to her skin, but still fierce with purpose. She gives up her crown, her glorious raiment, her lapis beads, her staff of power, her very sense of self. Inanna is killed by her sister, left hanging in the Underworld for seven days, and then is restored to life and transported back to the surface. The epic poem chronicles her journey of ascent and the reclamation of her power and self-agency in the realm above once more. The imagery lingers with me forever.

During my own workshop the next day, we paint plaster goddesses that I have prepared in scores and brought along to share with the other people at the retreat. I carefully paint a labyrinth on the belly of my goddess and around her neck I lay down a painted string of lapis beads.

Some years later I attend a birth art session at an ICAN conference (International Cesarean Awareness Network) with Pam England, midwife and author of *Birthing from Within,* who first popularized the use of the Inanna story with childbirth preparation. I am changed forever by her words:

*Where you were the most wounded—the place where the meat was **chewed off your bones**—becomes the seat of your most **powerful medicine** and the place where you can reach someone where no one else can.*

I call upon the story of Inanna during every pregnancy and childbirth experience and into other passages of womanhood and women's ritual as well. I find there are so many microcosmic journeys of descent and renewal present in each person's life: passages of initiation, of rebirth and re-making. I share these words with childbirth education clients and later with soldiers in the US military in the college classes I teach on the army base. I share them with women in the Red Tent.

Inanna's story and Persephone's story both remind us that there is a sweet nectar of joy in every rising sun, every raindrop and every petal. Both stories are medicine.

Interestingly, there is some evidence that there is a pre-Greek story of Persephone that also originates in Sumer. Though Inanna's story is first recorded 4000 years prior to Persephone's, the flavor of descent, initiation, renewal, and return to flourishing echo through both.

I think of them now, these goddesses stripped raw and shaking, descending deeper than they ever thought possible, frayed and worn and faltering, and yet still moving onward, step by step. Here I am stalled and fragile, worn and wondering, and for a moment I feel like an everyday Inanna, laying aside my power and confronting the darkness. I feel like Persephone, seeds of truth on my lips, the calls of weary souls ringing through me. Once, in an essay for *Feminism and Religion,* I wrote that in our own lives we face many Inanna's descents of our own. They may be as difficult as the death of an adult child, the loss of a baby, the diagnosis of significant illness, or a destroyed relationship. They may be as beautiful and yet soul-wrenchingly difficult as journeying through childbirth and walking through the Underworld of postpartum with our newborns. They may be as seemingly everyday as returning to school after a long absence. There is value in seeing our lives through this mythopoetic lens. When we story our realities, we find a connection to the experiences and courage of others, we find the pattern of our own lives, and we find a strength of purpose to go on.

I have called on Inanna in birthing and postpartum, I've called on her as I've led women from the Red Tent on a journey along a narrow riverbank seeking water from the sacred spring. I've called on her while picking raspberries with my children, our cheeks and hands streaked with red juice, crawling on our knees beneath thorny brambles in search of our treasure. Now, sitting on my back deck, my wounded leg extended in front of me, I extend myself out to Persephone, she of shadowed places and unknown spaces. She knows what it is like to be stranded and alone.

> *Persephone,*
> *please walk with me,*
> *in tender fierceness,*
> *bold stillness,*
> *deliberate action,*
> *brave love,*
> *and sacred truth.*
> *Please guide me*
> *through the Underworld*
> *of confusion and despair*
> *and out into the sunshine*

where compassion,
joy,
and devotion
can blossom into fullness.

Cut Off

I feel cut off from Mark, our nightly walks in which we explore and talk together, have abruptly ended. Those conversations, those steps, shape our relationship, our connection to one another as whole and complex and interesting people. Now we snatch moments of conversation over the heads of children, but there is no shared delight in noticing and experiencing the world together.

When I'm outside, I feel tender, vulnerable, at risk, instead of alert, connected, in tune, and expansive. *I see why animals who hurt their legs often die,* I tell Mark.

The peace of the woods feels distant and uncertain. I feel aimless, forcibly separated from my soul-fuel, my place of nourishment. The challenge here, I know, is to find new places within myself, instead of with my body, but also perhaps within my own dark and cluttered home.

We built our house by hand, but it is dim inside due to the thick straw bale walls with relatively small windows set into two-foot-thick walls. The possessions of six people and a business have stretched its capacity until it feels like a heap of matter, a site of projects in flux, abandoned ideas, plans, projects.

There is so much that needs tending that I don't have time to tend, so much that needs care, when my care is frayed and thin. I need to marshal my other resources, muster my reserves, dig deep, restructure and review. This *is* the work. I am doing it. Maybe it is time to open my arms to really being *here,* to making my home a place of respite and peace, instead of fleeing for the solitude of the woods. I'm not sure what I can reach out to, or where the Goddess lives if not in green places and wild spaces. I feel silenced and alone. I need to find new ways to connect and listen. New ways to trust. I also need to trust my body, my bones and muscles as they repair themselves in this magical way of being human.

I will trust the process, trust the progress, trust the book and keep watching it all unfold in beautiful, capable, and inspiring ways. It is all I can do: keep going, keep noticing, keep telling, keep being here. *I don't have to figure anything out,* that isn't the point and has never been the point. This is witnessing space. That's what it is and what I'm doing: living into witnessing, living into the story as it unfolds, leaving a margin for magic, making room for rest, listening, listening, listening.

How do I keep going when I'm so forcibly grounded?

Sit with what is. This is the cauldron now. Seeing what you can see.

Yesterday, I listened to my own past audio recording about finding your lost magic. In it, I first suggest thinking about the things you need to fuel your own magic and then making sure you are doing them. I suggest cleaning out stale altar spaces, putting away books you aren't reading, decks you aren't using, tools you aren't exploring. Then, I suggest changing something, either trying something new, or revisiting something old. Picking up a practice that you've abandoned, or trying a fresh one. I also suggest, paradoxically, either "going big" or "going small." By going small, I mean committing to something extremely simple, simplifying your practices down to the very basics. Or, going big, planning an elaborate personal ceremony of dedication and vows-renewal for example, dressing up making special foods, really going "all in," to a ritual of reclamation and renewal.

I suddenly wonder if this is my opportunity, my time, to begin a dedicated devotional practice indoors, to Persephone. This may be the moment, the action, I've been waiting for. I can intensify my study of her, dialog with her, consciously engage and dig more deeply. I easily connect to nature, Gaia, the goddess of woodspaces and open places. *Where might I connect within the walls of my home, reaching out with my mind and heart?*

> *Who am I*
> *when I'm not trying to fix myself?*
> Shh, the wise grandmother-self whispers
> *only you know the story*
> *of this spider*
> *and how it walks through the air.*

Summer Solstice

I wake with the Solstice sun, slicing briefly through the window between green branches. By the time I go out to sit on the deck in the morning, gray clouds have descended and far-off thunder rumbles. The hawk calls briefly and then falls silent. A yellow bird hops from milkweed to raspberry and back again. I think about how I am trying to force an answer, a response, a next step. Am I trying to push for more? What if I try an extremely radical acceptance of exactly what is? Into the quiet, slowness of the gray sky, the hawk begins to call again, just for a few minutes.

I start to sing quietly to myself. I sing my Persephone prayersong, my sun and bones song, and my own holy text songs. It feels good to put them together, to sing things that I've written over the last three months, on this mostly invisible journey into the reclamation of my soul.

Is today the day, I wonder, *when my work with Persephone will be done?* It is Summer Solstice, we have traveled together for three months. *Is this the time when she will pull away, now that the earth is restored to flourishing?* When I originally committed to Persephone, drinking my pomegranate juice, making my offering, and promising my devotion, garnet bracelet on my wrist, I'd said I would work with her for three months. Here I am, three months in, and there is still so much more to uncover. Persephone's story is not simple, her journey is complex and multi-layered. I was wrong to think I could tie things up into a neat box, lessons learned, soul healed, life rewoven in only three months.

Instead of continuing to ask for a sign from the goddess, I just wait.

> *Persephone,*
> *I offer you three breaths…*
> *one from my center*
> *one from my heart*
> *one from my mind.*
> *I am open to your guidance.*
> *I am open to what is.*

My eyes are closed, head tilted back as I offer my breaths, this first step in a daily devotional practice. For a few brief moments, the sun emerges and warms my closed eyelids. A breeze lifts my hair and caresses my face. Then, clouds cover the sun, my leg aches against the weathered boards of the deck.

I open to the day's page in my *Desire Map* planner. *Devotion cures,* it says at the bottom of the page. My walk with Persephone has been a walk of devotion. Being stilled and recovering requires devotion too. *Devotion heals,* I might say.

Solstice afternoon, the sky grows dark and the trees begin to bend and sway. Heavy rain begins and then hail falls, the size of marbles, skittering across the porch and whipping my red roses. I can hardly believe it is the midpoint of the year already. In purple ink across a white page, I write a summer blessing for our community:

> *May you tilt your face to the sky*
> *and receive a warm blessing from the sun.*
> *May you open your arms to the moon*
> *and take a long drink of summer moonbeams.*
> *May you sing with the river's flow*
> *and dance with the fairies and your dreams.*
> *May you wreath your days with smiles,*
> *soak in streams of enchantment,*
> *know delight in your footsteps,*
> *and courage in your heart.*
> *May you know blooming.*
> *May you know blessing.*
> *May you know deep wells of peace.*

I put on a purple dress and place a crown of flowers on my hair. I collect my small children, we make our way out into the cloud-dark rain to go to my sister-in-law's house for Solstice fairy tea party with the cousins.

The table is laden with fairy lights and jewels and tea cups are arrayed at each place. We eat miniature biscuits with homemade hedgerow jelly, lemon cupcakes with raspberry mascarpone frosting, and tiny brownie brownies as we drink ginger peach tea. Afterwards, we pool our resources and make fairy terrariums, bright green moss layered in glass jars with imitation butterflies, bird's eggs, and other small trinkets and treasures arrayed around the edges.

After dinner, we gather for our simple family Summer Solstice ritual. I originally planned to circle outside during sunset, mystical trails of incense drifting
in the humid air as we created a flower mandala together. But it is overcast and
drizzling. The little kids suggest a footbath ritual instead, and so we circle our
chairs between the kitchen and living room, filling tubs of hot water and passing
ritual salts, oils, and dried flowers around to one another. I decide to step outside
briefly into the light spattering of raindrops and pick one Queen Anne's Lace
blossom for each person as well as a handful of rose petals. The flowers are completely prone, weighed down with rain. As I look at the flowers, I see the wild,
spontaneous, unconstrained magic within them and some words of blessing trail
through my mind, *May you make your own magic out of weeds and wonder.* This
is what we do, weaving a sort of tapestry of everyday sorcery through our very
normal lives. Inside, we each hold our flower briefly, tenderly, and offer a wish
for the second half of the year, before we let it drop into our footbath container.
We offer blessings to one another and sing together in our dimly lit room, a
candle on the floor in the center of us and incense drifting lazily through the
evening air.

Letting Go

There are two bright red birds in the mulberry tree when I wake up. The deck is
strewn with fallen leaves and small oak branches after yesterday's storm.

I sit in a chair looking out at the gray sky through the green branches. It is
heavy and overcast again. The hawk calls once, twice, three times. I place one
hand on my belly and one hand on my heart and offer three breaths to morning,
to Persephone, to the Goddess and I open myself to what is. This is the small
devotional practice I am committing to while I continue to recover from my
ankle injury. I am amazed by the impact of offering three conscious, intentional
breaths. Once again, the sun breaks briefly through the clouds to touch my eyelids as I finish my words and the wind swirls up my arms and across my shoulders. I am not saying that the weather is responding to me or is being controlled
for me on my behalf, but regardless of objective reality and weather patterns, it
still feels as if my breaths have been received and responded to.

I sit for a few moments, in presence, my hand on my heart and the other hand on my belly and I feel a wave of tenderness for myself, similar to the tenderness I felt for the women at Red Tent when we lifted one another's bodies.

Let go, I whisper softly to the gray sky. *Be with what is, right now.*

But what am I to let go of? Persephone? Has our time together come to an end?

I sit in the tenderness for a moment, wondering what it would feel like to be tender with myself more often, to greet my life with tenderness as often as I can.

Who am I without my sadness? Without my connections? Without my pain?

Who am I, alone in the rain?

I sit quietly with my hand on my heart, not wanting to leave the three breaths of presence.

Shh...

Place one hand on your wild heart

What does she have to say?

Listen.

Stepping into Magic

One day you will find yourself
teetering at the brink
forked tongue tasting the air
and eyes full of fire.
It is good to be alive and breathing
on the precipice of change.

I wake this morning with these words in my head, persistent, insistent, rolling around and around and around. For the first time in days, there is a bright slice of morning sunlight shining through the bedroom window. I try to say my morning prayers as I always do before getting up, but the *forked tongue tasting*

the air continues to roll through my mind and I feel compelled to get up and write it down immediately, before continuing my prayers during toothbrushing instead of pre-rising.

I step out onto the sunny deck with my tea in hand. I make a slow circuit, hearing and then spotting a phoebe high in the top branches, calling to morning under a waning moon.

This is the real work, I think, *sitting in the sun with a cup of tea, learning how to rest.* Then, I think of all the other work of the world and wonder if sitting with tea is an indulgence, a privilege denied to many, a spoiled type of living. I think of all the other real work, holding the children, sweeping the floor, fulfilling the orders. *It is **all** the real work,* I think, *and the question truly is: can you carry a calm heart into the swirling center of so much life?*

I breathe deep, sun spangling my eyelashes and making me squint as I watch for the hawk in the segments of blue sky visible between branches. I place my hand on my belly and offer my three breaths of presence to Persephone, to morning. I sit with my eyes closed briefly, thinking—though I try to avoid making "bargains"—about how what I see or think next after taking these breaths feels like a sign, a message, a communication, an answer. I open my eyes and within three beats, I see a shadow. I assume it is the vulture again, but instead a beautiful great blue heron crests the treetops and glides slowly across the sky right in front of me, strong, steady wing beats carrying it gracefully away before my grateful eyes. I think about how these sightings and experiences don't *have* to mean anything specific, it is enough to just *live them,* to be alert and interested in the world, and to feel glad to be here to *see it.*

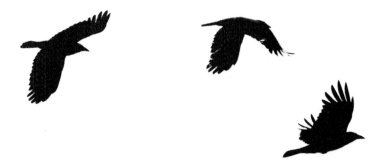

After the workday is over, I step outside into the late afternoon sun to take some photos for a shop listing. I hear a crow immediately, then see another crow swoop low through the treetops, followed almost immediately by a third. The hawk cries out. I feel happy, surprised, and pleased by this little gift, this moment of magic, just waiting for me and I wonder what else I've missed cooped up indoors. What are the chances that I would step out and into magic immediately, every time I open the back door?

I go to step back inside of this very same door, when I startle and let out a cry of surprise, for there, stretched completely across the length of the threshold is a languid black snake. I cannot believe my eyes. I know I must have stepped right over it, oblivious, on my way out the door, and I almost stepped back over it, unseeing, right now.

As I watch, its forked tongue tastes the air, and my morning message echoes once more through my mind. I can hardly believe it, this connection feels so visceral, so surprising, so meaningful, so real. I remember my wondering from a few weeks if I could even stand it, could even manage to hold any more astonishment about the real-life magic of the world, how I have to pace myself so as not to be overwhelmed by the flood of enchantment.

The snake is motionless, shiny and black with a small amount of white lining the underside of its head and belly. It stares, black-eyed, tongue flickering and then begins to move, sinuous and languid. It moves about two feet away from the back door, in a precise line where the porch meets the exterior wall and then suddenly doubles back on itself, gliding back across the threshold and away the opposite direction, sliding along the porch line, against the foundation and out of sight.

I show Mark the lines I felt so compelled to write down this morning. *I could not make this stuff up!* I exclaim with glee.

I think about the snake, remembering its position along the threshold, a literal threshold moment for me. I realize the world has offered me my own ceremony of transition, built it for me, right in front of my eyes.

Medusa is here!

I'm not sure why it has taken me so long to see it, but I feel like I suddenly understand that I don't have to lay aside my work with Persephone or with Air to move into also working with Medusa and Earth. It isn't about "switching," it is about adding to and deepening. I feel the sweep and curl of air around me, sliding up my feet and around my shoulders.

> *Imagine what might happen if you laid aside*
> *the planning and the proving,*
> *the pushing and pursuing,*

and stepped into the ceremonies Life
is weaving right outside your door,
before your eyes,
under your skin.

Medusa

I lie down and offer my breaths. The air stirs up briefly, stroking me, but I feel a certain sensation of disconnect and longing.

I try to compose a new prayer, perhaps one for Medusa, but I feel dull and lacking in inspiration and the words don't come. I need time and focus, space and opportunity, not a cramped slice of morning on a wooden deck with someone riding a bike in circles around my head.

Medusa, please rise through me.

When Medusa spoke to or through me last year, she said:

I *am alive*
and I *am powerful.*
If you dare to
shed your skin
and meet my eyes
you will see yourself
reflected there.
Wholly whole.
Unbound.
Soft
and angry.

My thoughts return to anger: women's anger, maternal anger, humanitarian anger, rage, despair... Anger can paralyze us, we might even fear that expressing our rage could freeze others, and so it seeps out in small ways, snaking through our communications with those we hold most dear. *Do I feel permitted to express anger?* I wonder. *Am I frozen by, with, or within my own rage?*

The anthology published by The Girl God, *Re-visioning Medusa,* explores the cultural, social, political, and religious significance of Medusa's story and how it has been presented, particularly as it relates to women's justifiable rage. It also describes Medusa's herstorical roots as a powerful older goddess from Libya.

> *I saw you once, Medusa;*
> *we were alone.*
> *I looked you straight in the cold eye, cold.*
> *I was not punished,*
> *was not turned to stone.*
> *How to believe the legends I am told?*
> *...I turned your face around!*
> *It is my face.*
> *That frozen rage is what I must explore*
> *—Oh secret, self-enclosed,*
> *and ravaged place!*
> *That is the gift I thank Medusa for.*

> **—May Sarton, "The Muse as Medusa", quoted in *Re-Visioning Medusa* by The Girl God**

In the patriarchal Medusa story, Medusa is assaulted in the goddess temple where she serves Athena. When she dares to respond with rage, she is punished and destroyed, though her head—snake-haired and wild—still has the power to destroy men with a single glance. Medusa both frightens and intrigues me. I do not feel like I've truly ever really been allowed to be angry, but the anger is there, bubbling below the surface. *How would it feel to let indignation and rage and fierce passion rise up through me, no longer swallowing feelings as too big or bold or not allowed?*

Medusa was refashioned by her attackers as a monster, someone who deserved to die for her rage, for her feelings, for her power. As with many Greek myths, Medusa existed long before the Greeks got their hands on her tale and shifted her myth to suit their purposes and reinforce their lessons for Greek women. Medusa was one of three aspects of a Libyan triple goddess, Anatha, the Amazon tribes in these areas known as "Gorgons." This Medusa was known as a serpent goddess, a sea goddess, and a sun goddess. She was a goddess of wisdom and dark mysteries, a goddess of divination, healing, and renewal. It can be difficult to piece together accurate stories from the slender remaining evidence, but like Persephone—and many other ancient goddesses—Medusa was simplified, de-radicalized, and weakened in the stories that appear after patriarchal culture rose to dominance and supplanted the Goddess with their own tales.

Medusa, please rise through me.
Help me to know my own strength,
taste my own courage,
dance with determination.
Let me not shy away from my skills,
not turn away from my talents,
but let me turn to face them,
eyes full of flame,
and resolve formed of stone.

Rose Lessons

There is no late, there is just what is, and that's okay. This is what I realize as I step outside with my tea and stack of journals this morning, wishing I'd gotten up earlier, wondering what has happened to the time. The clouds are white puffs in the blue sky, sun filtering through the trees, and a thin layer of sweat already forming rapidly on my upper lip. My attention is caught by the rosebush, the blooms rich and fresh and abundant. They have re-righted themselves after having been borne low by rain. I gather some petals from flowers that are about to drop and put them in a soft pile by my journals.

As I sit with my rose, rose hips, and rose petals, a memory of an older poem drifts back to me:

> *She prays,*
> *hopes,*
> *and heals*
> *in roses.*
> *This is the season*
> *of rose prayers.*
> *Witnessing,*
> *celebrating,*
> *honoring,*
> *offering.*

I have loved roses since I was twenty years old and planted a red rosebush in the backyard of my college duplex building. I would sit by the roses in the afternoon, watching the butterflies, feeling the sun, the busy atmosphere of a large university town melting away. I remember feeling aware of my connection to the very life force of the universe, embodied in these brilliant red blooms. I had one of my first "religious experiences," sitting by this rose, suddenly becoming viscerally aware of the current of life itself, the sacred, winding through the world.

Now, each year, at my home in the woods, the roses rise again each spring, blooming wildly and madly from April until November. I have tried other varieties of more elaborate roses, rather than the standard shrubs readily available at gardening shops, but it is the "double knock-out" shrub roses that flourish for me, bright and bountiful, lifting their red faces to the sun and wind. I have come to associate them with Persephone, she who brings the spring, who brings the blossoming, who brings renewal and rebirth, who causes the earth and our lives to burst into bloom once more.

I think about religion in general, how so many people seem to be looking for the one right truth, a crutch, something to make it all better or something that promises to fix everything or yourself. Goddess, for me, has always been a soft place to land, a comfort, a welcoming presence, but maybe it is time to let her rise up through me, active, dynamic, passionate, even angry. I remember something I just heard Jennifer Louden say in The Oasis, perhaps paraphrasing Thomas Merton "Sometimes we don't actually need to rest, we need to find our own inspiration."

Looking up at the sun striped trees, I suddenly become filled with awareness that while I feel like I am allowed to live among them and feel intense gratitude for that, I protect them also. We are all part of so many systems of degradation that it is powerful to recognize that which I do so thoroughly and with such love. Maybe I don't need more tenderness, I think, maybe I need more fierceness.

Maybe you need both.

Medusa and Persephone are both tender to begin with and become fierce through necessity, maturity, and determination. I am tender now and rising into fierceness.

I've been unraveling my life and I'm not sure when it is time to focus on re-weaving, reknitting, and strengthening. Earth is an element is for stabilizing and grounding, and now, with my injured ankle holding me firmly to the ground, I think this is where I am, the point to which I have traveled, the perspective and lessons I have now to learn.

The hawk cries out and I notice that all the leaves in front of me are glowing. I start to sing an elemental invocation song, drawing the words out of memory and re-stringing them together. A chant for Hecate floats to mind as well and I sing it briefly too. A shadow rises overhead and so swiftly I almost miss it, a crow swoops over my shoulder and into the woods, cawing.

> *This is the season of rose prayers,*
> *the soft and beautiful,*
> *the hopeful and heroic,*
> *the gifts that lift tender hearts*
> *to meet the sun,*
> *weaving light into life.*
> *There is wind in my hair,*
> *the light touch of both petals*
> *and thorns beneath my fingertips,*
> *a softening in my heart*
> *as it cracks open anew*

beneath a faded moon,
a misty sky,
a whisper of longing,
a blush of renewal,
a quiet promise
of delicate dreams in bloom,
the deep roots of desire,
and the grounding work
of blossoming.
Here we are
rooted and rising
from the depths of
a wondering earth.

You Are Healing

I wake this morning concerned about what feels like growing stiffness and lack of mobility in my ankle joint. Though I am up early, instead of going out to the deck, I sit in the living room watching physical therapy and rehabilitation videos and getting Mark to rub my tender ankle and foot. After carefully studying the video, he uses his broad hands to manually push one of my leg bones back and, while cringing a bit, I feel an instant difference. While I am a long way from fully healed, I feel encouraged by this change and feel more confidently aware that, with time and attention, I will fully recover.

I turn the page in my planner to today's page and smile to see the words printed along the bottom like a promise:

You are healing.

I reflect that because of the attention paid to the events of each day this year, this may be one of the most memorable years of my life, even though it is a totally normal, average, humdrum sort of year and yet, somehow, at the same time, so full of magic, mystery, enchantment, beauty, and wonder that I can barely contain it all. The intensity, connections, and interweavings are so numerous and rich.

My daily meditation for today in *Simple Abundance* reads:

Life accidents prune us back. Our souls become broken fields, plowed by pain.

Sarah Ban Breathnach goes on to note that she knows intellectually that pruning strengthens rather than weakens, but that this seems counterintuitive,

> *...pruning is necessary for complete growth. So, I have come to realize, is a certain amount of pain in our lives. Pain prunes the unessential emotions, ambitions, and illusions, teaching us the lessons we either consciously or unconsciously refuse to be taught by joy. Pain prunes the insignificant details that distract us from what is really important, sapping our days, energies, and spirits... If we don't prune away the stress and plow under the useless in our lives, pain will do it for us.*

I know many people cope with chronic illnesses. I have several myself, including a chronic pain disorder (currently in remission) and this thought from Sarah is by no means meant to blame the victim or to suggest that pains are visited on us due to incorrect thinking patterns, or consciously, willfully imposed on us by grander powers than our own in order to teach us "lessons." Those modes of thought and lines of thinking are damaging and insidious. She goes on to explain:

> *Make no mistake, I think pain is a wretched gardener. Her cuts stun and sting. But after pruning, preferably voluntary, we're able to discern what's real, what's important, what's essential for our happiness. Be of good cheer. Study your plants and study your lifestyle. When the right time arrives, go into the garden with sharp shears. Speak kindly. Pray softly. Prune back. Now plow ahead.*

I recognize a persistent sensation of worry that I have been "wasting" days, not doing as much as I could or should be doing. Finally, sitting in bed typing after reading, writing, playing and reflecting, I recognize once more that what I am feeling is the unfamiliar state of not having "too much to do." It is an uncomfortable sensation, actually. Being overdone and worn is such a usual state that not being so registers as discomfort or as something "wrong." This is something that is key for me to continue to be aware of.

Looking Back

I wake thinking of ancestry and family stories, of the countries and lands from which my DNA has wound its way through thousands upon thousands of years, lives, and generations.

I get out my grandmother's family history book, looking for the names of my maternal line that have slipped my mind since I used to pour through the book in childhood, naming families of small toys after these not-too-distant ancestors. I am reading a book about mitochondrial DNA *(The Seven Daughters of Eve* by Bryan Sykes*)* and it has prompted me to go exploring my lineage. I end up perusing my journals from twenty years ago that are stored in the same box. They are frustrating in their lack of detail, their repetitiveness, their endless musings turning over the same three or four questions. While I still feel like the "same person," I also like myself better now. I am more solid in my skin, happier, more well-rounded, more well-informed, more thoughtful, less self-centered, more secure, deeper, more spiritually rooted.

Are we realer when we're alone or together? I wonder. *Are our inner lives, our rolling thoughts, the stuff of a genuinely whole life, or is the wholeness woven in our webs of interconnection and relationships, our connections and experiences with one another, sharing life, not alone and witnessing?*

Potluck at my parents' house this afternoon is in honor of Mark's birthday: he is forty-two. I met him before his seventeenth birthday. Time is such a strange and miraculous thing. I have used ten eggs and four sticks of butter to make his favorite cake: German chocolate. The kids swim and Mark grills bratwursts for the family while my sister makes frozen butterbeer drinks for everyone.

As everyone talks and visits, I recognize the same sensation of feeling most alive and genuine, most real, when alone. My inner world is rich with connection that feels stifled or silenced when in the company of others, even those beloved to me. My dad and I talk briefly about ancestry and genetics, him telling me that a segment of our ancestors traveled from France to settle in Canada in the 1600s and then made their way to Missouri in the oldest colony on this side of the Mississippi. I tell him that after poking around this I've found information about my maternal grandfather's side down to Plymouth.

In reading *The Seven Daughters of Eve* I find myself humbled to my bones to expand my sense of ancestry and identity across thousands of years instead of hundreds. How many stories intersecting? *How many lives have been lived? How many triumphs and tragedies in the genetic unwinding and pathwork that have eventually led to this moment?*

JULY

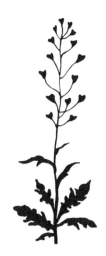

Kindling

I worry that with so much casting off and shedding, I might be losing some of my own fire, putting out my flames. My enthusiasm for, or enjoyment of, things I used to enjoy doing seems to be dimming. Or, is it just simplifying, clarifying, and finally, at long last, discerning the difference between could do and want to, shoulds and desires? Are these becoming more cleanly and clearly differentiated? On warm mornings under blue skies, it seems likely. On late nights after not "getting it all done," I still wonder.

I am definitely laying things aside this year and there is space now between responsibilities to potentially pick some things back up. Or not. I wonder if I have cultivated a growing disinterest in them that cannot be rekindled. *Do I want to rekindle anything? What do I need to feed my flame? When is stoking a blaze unnecessary and I can instead sit in a cool breeze, doing nothing?*

All I know, is that I feel an actual easing in my shoulders and around my heart when I think of how much I had been carrying that I've now laid down.

Working in the tiny temple, I hear an insight wandering into my brain: *Just trust. Notice and respond. That is really all you need to do.*

Maybe it is possible to just trust myself, the rhythm of the days, the ebb and flow of inspiration, the natural, continued unfolding of my life as it occurs, step by step, day by day, breath by breath.

We all need white spaces in our lives,
our books,
our days,
our hearts,
the world.
Margins,
edges,
buffers,
borders,
boundaries.
Expanses of softness and silence that stretch
to soothe the eye and restore the soul.
Spaces that mute
the swift and busy
and sparkle with
promise
in the sun.

Sunset at New Moon

I feel an urge to get outside quickly this morning, in case I am missing something. I leave my tea to steep and step out into already humid and stifling air. The hawks are calling already, distantly.

My roses have all been devoured by Japanese beetles, their neon red beauty destroyed, beetles nestled in their shredded hearts. One rose appears to be whole, but it is too far down for me to reach from the deck and I feel resistant to stepping down off the porch on my still unstable ankle. I make my slow circuits around the deck, stepping carefully and as close to normally as possible and realize that I feel uneasy and scared almost about returning to my daily visits to the woods, as if I have become "at risk" there, vulnerable instead of safe. These gray boards and twining greenery have become my new sanctuary. Blackberry canes have worked their way through one corner of the deck, forming a wild little patch above the boards that delights me with its persistence.

I think about devotion and building new devotional practices. I brainstorm a list of the devotional practices I could begin, deepen, or continue, for Persephone, for Medusa, for both, for the incomprehensible Goddess I feel as a whole, woven around and through the entire world and out into the swirling cosmos. My own past poem about the new moon floats through my mind, only partially remembered. When I go in to look it up, I'm interested to see that I last shared it in the context of one of my own past audio recordings about devotion and renewal. There is something here to pay attention to, I can feel it, waiting to be noticed.

> *Sunset at new moon*
> *laid down a path*
> *across the flowers,*
> *twilight shadowed*
> *sun sparkles*
> *whispering*
> *of a knowing*
> *that requests patient*
> *listening,*
> *and a wondering*
> *that will kiss your dreams*
> *tonight.*
> *Remembering*
> *how in timeless*
> *shadows,*
> *you hear the yes*
> *carried*
> *on the wind.*

It is so warm today, that I don't go back outside. Instead, I create my new moon collage goddess, reconfiguring one of my poems into the words that twine along her edges and fill her center with truth:

It is good to be alive and breathing, teetering on the brink, forked tongue tasting the air, and eyes full of fire. You live a miracle every day and you don't have to earn it.

I choose my oracle cards for the month and catch up with my monthly goal planning page. I have the first headache that I've had in almost a full month and feel dull and pinched as I push through it to write on my pages anyway.

Recognizing the sensation I take an ibuprofen, rather than willing myself to get better without one.

I had meant to write and think about devotion, about devotional practices, and perhaps build some practices to implement tomorrow, but I don't feel it. While some writers write of doing it anyway, of just putting the pen to the page, of not giving up, of dragging the writing out of you, I find in my own life that inspiration is rarely a problem and that I do not lack capacity to motivate myself, or drive myself forward. Instead, what I lack too often, is the patience to let myself sit without driving, to soften into the arms of the wind, and to let go of the rope instead of dragging. Sometimes, that actually might mean letting inspiration fly past me and watching it go, trusting in its capacity to rise again within me tomorrow, an infinite wellspring of creative power and indwelling joy.

Stepping outside, I have come to realize, is my signal to move into "writer's mind," where my senses all become alert for the next part of the story. I wonder if I could enter into it at other times and in other places, not only waiting for the balm of the outdoors to settle into my bones and skin, switching me on.

In Natalie Goldberg's *Writing Down the Bones*, she writes:

> *Our lives are at once ordinary and mythical. We live and die. [...] Our lives are important, magnificent really, and their details are worthy to be recorded. This is how writers must think, this is how we must sit down with pen in hand. We were here; we are human beings; this is how we lived. Let it be known, the earth passed before us. Our details are important. Otherwise, if they are not, we can drop a bomb and it doesn't matter.*

It is my own understanding of this magnificence—the everyday magic, ordinary mysteries, and powerful mundanity of our lives—that guides and shapes this book and this moment for me. You have a choice to see things as mattering, as having meaning, or as not mattering or having no meaning. Either way, you are right.

The fireflies are already blinking above ironweed buds and elderflowers. Just the smallest hint of pink-orange touches a few clouds and lingers in one deep orange stripe behind the trees. One determined hawk continues to shriek persistently over the treetops even though darkness is falling rapidly. I glance up to see a perfect slender silver sickle of new moon hanging framed by the branches of two tall oak trees. The eerie sound of coyotes howling begins to rise into the spaces between fireworks and thunder.

A Month

It has been exactly one month since I fell. The remaining roses by the deck are frosted with silver dew. There are lightning bugs nestled asleep under curled mulberry leaves. The hawks are awake, high and distant, repetitive and constant, like an arcade game shooting through the silence. There is an unfamiliar taste of coolness in the air and for a moment I almost think of fall. A breeze curls around my elbows and moves my hair and a cicada creaks in the cedars. A few more puffs of purple have appeared atop the ironweed and I hear two crows cawing briefly, opposite the hawks. I wonder if I've been getting outside too late for the crows, if they've already swept by before I step my weary, slow feet upon these slats of board.

I wonder what would happen if I decided to stop writing now. *How would I draw my conclusion, share my final thoughts? What would I say and what have I learned?*

I lie back with my head by the blackberry leaves to offer my three breaths to Persephone.

I was worried I lost my thread, but I realize that I haven't, I just changed my habits briefly to a pattern that didn't prioritize the unwinding. Somehow, with lots of slow steps and unrelenting practice, I've become a writer. I had to wiggle and stretch and affirm and grow into social work, into motherhood, into birthwork, into teaching, into priestessing, and now, here, finally, I am wiggling and stretching and growing into what I've been meant to be all along.

> *Keeping getting up*
> *in the morning.*
> *Keep loving the way*
> *the sun shines.*
> *Keep being surprised*
> *and delighted*
> *by the landscape of colors*
> *as the wheel turns.*
> *Keep looking for birds,*
> *for they carry magic*
> *across the sky right to your eyes.*
> *Listen for moonlight.*
> *Turn your head when*

you hear a branch crack.
Talk to crows.
Spend time with hawks.
Converse with wild berries of all kinds
for they hold whole
fields of possibility
beneath their skins.
If rain falls, let it soak.
Laugh with the thunder.
Whisper prayers
and promises to the wind.
Cry under rainbows.
Sing to clouds.
And let the wildflowers
of the roadsides
teach you what it means to live.

Community

The day is incredibly hot and humid as we gather for our first Family Tent event. The women of Red Tent and their families have been invited to an all-day retreat and river day. We circle together awkwardly for a simple opening ritual. It is difficult to expect instant connection or ritual collaboration with a multi-age, multi-gender group, many of whom have never met one another or circled together before. We manage though, standing in the clover underneath spreading oak and sycamore trees, holding hands and singing under the broad blue sky.

The highlight of the day for me is our Orange Tent event for boys ages two to ten. Tanner named it Orange Tent after spending his whole life hearing about Red Tent and Pink Tent. I do like how Orange (like Pink) has its origin source in Red. Orange is also a fiery, warm, and energetic color, much like the passion, drive, and energy of many little boys. We set up a canopy and drape orange fabric from the sides. In the center, I lay an orange Triple Moon altar cloth. Mark collects fresh water from the spring in a clear glass bowl and we float orange candles in the bowl.

During our circle, the boys take turns lighting the floating candles and then hold pinches of bright calendula petals in their hands, warming them, and then making an offering or wish into the clear spring water. My heart is full seeing them sitting in circle together, little legs folded, energetic eyes, faces, and voices participating in their first sacred circle together as a group. Three fathers and three mothers participate as well. Tanner was very emphatic that Orange Tent was for all people, not just boys. We drum and sing and talk about our own "hero's heart" inspired by Melia Keeton-Digby's book, *The Hero's Heart,* and how each person can be a hero, it doesn't have to involve strength or toughness or special powers, it can involve kindness and helpfulness and everyday gestures of friendship.

We sing a modified version of a song by Shining Wheel Pagan Chorus:

We are children of the earth
we are one and the same
we are connected to the web
we are part of the chain.

These are our sons, earnest and eager to connect with one another, with us, with the magic of our world. They are just as capable of sitting in circle and sharing their experiences as our girls, if we allow them space to do so. After our song and drum game, we carve soap with plastic knives into a heart or other heroic symbol. We paint wooden suns that Mark has made for the boys and then paint power sticks to which we tie orange ribbons for them to run with under the sun. The fathers, small boys on their laps or sitting near them, paint together and as I watch them, heads bent together, I feel I have done truly good work on this day.

Later, we make foraged saining wands and my heart fills again to see Tanner sitting at the table with Mark, earnestly bundling up his cedar, yarrow, and vervain. This is family magic.

The container for ceremony feels "leaky" as the day wears on, and people come and go. It feels energetically chaotic and hard for me to manage on a personal level. The day is long and heavy and hot and I wish we would have planned a shorter event. The responsibility for holding the energy, for planning for and satisfying the needs and interests of so many people, feels like an oppressive weight. We end up at the pavilion for a full ten hours, a long time to be outdoors in the July humidity and a long time to sustain a nourishing spiritual experience for other people and tending to my own children while still teetering on an uncertain ankle.

My head begins to throb as I get home, reviewing the details with Mark in a sun-slowed recitation of what went well, what didn't go well, what we could have done differently. Despite the high point joy of the Orange Tent portion of the day, I am short-tempered and irritable, agitated by things like people not bringing plates or food for dinner, even though I asked them to several times. We agree that perhaps we should have concluded shortly after lunch, just held Orange Tent, or just had a river afternoon with a potluck dinner. Trying to do everything at once was overkill. This is not the first time I've had the same lesson. I wonder when or if it will ever stick.

When do we push ourselves, and when do we grant ourselves grace, or a moment of understanding, a pass?

This is one of my reflections on the group dynamics of Red Tent as well, our self-care, our honoring of ourselves, our limits, capacities, availability, and so on:

When is it self-kindness to drop the ball, so to speak, and when is it an unfair burden to place on the rest of the group to have you not fulfill your commitment, to show up unprepared and expect others to fill in the gaps left by the things you forgot, left behind, or excused yourself from (often in the name of self-care)?

When do you show up, looking for a community to sustain you, to give to you, to nourish you, without offering anything in return?

When do you make remarks about lacking community, wanting to build community, or wanting to find community, while seemingly oblivious to your own role in giving to that community which you seek?

It is not always about what you can take, what can feed you, or what your soul needs to flourish and thrive, because you do not exist in vacuum, and the communities that exist do not do so in order to serve you, but with an expectation that you will participate in the life and health of that community, even if it sometimes isn't convenient to you personally.

Communities rely on energy to fuel and sustain them, they are collaborative endeavors of commitment, devotion, action, and growth. The balance is difficult to assess—the need to care for yourself and to act in your own interests is important, and is something women are often actively, or biologically in the years of intensively nourishing children, socialized away from doing. However, the building of community is *collaborative* and something that requires devotion, focus, and a prioritizing of group health over personal whims. The container, the community, will not always be there to hold you, if you are not an active part of building its structure and taking your turn to hold others as well.

Breath by Breath

I wake early to a room bright-gold with sunrise. In my head, breezy and insistent, are the words: *be brave in protecting the margins of your blue-sky days.* Related thoughts begin to pour in about other people crowding into your white spaces, filling in all your margins for you. They are—ironically—quickly erased by the voices of my children, clamoring for roller skates to be put on, asking questions about homeschool co-op classes, and chatting about their lives. I feel restless and like I'm missing something, losing something important. Here I am without margin for my own thoughts, my own brain space, above the noises of home.

My mind drifts to my younger self. *Was she more fun, more interesting, more connected to herself? Did she laugh more before she became so encumbered by never-ending ideas, wants, and to-dos?*

By the time I toast waffles for the kids, make my tea, and do my physical therapy exercises for my ankle, it is mid-morning, my morning insights thready and faded. The day is already so hot when I step outside, that it instantly saps my life force, diminishes my energy, bringing the sensation of being stale and faded. I welcome the silence of the outdoors though, the solitude, the perspective, the potential to see something surprising. I begin to make my circuits on the still-wet boards, feeling bored and dull, like there is nothing new left to explore. Shadows of butterflies flutter just out of range above my head as I walk, wild grapevine twines briefly around my toes. There is a rustling sound in the leaves on the deck by the side of the house and I look to see a slender blue-tailed skink emerge and sit, watchfully on the brown leaves. A creaking cascade of bugsong rises in a wave of sound, rising in pitch and then ebbing away to silence.

I sing my Persephone song as I walk, slow paces on damp boards, clouds drifting in front of the sun and bringing a short reprieve from the relentless heat. As I finish my song, the sharp sound of a hawk rises directly in front of me, three times, and then stops. I can't help but feel answered, responded to, in these moments.

I read back through my words over the last four months, worried, as I have often been, that there is "nothing here." As I read, a storm kicks up, yellow leaves start to fly by the windows, the trees bend, and thunder rumbles overhead. Finally, the skies open and the rain pours down. I step out the front door onto the narrow front porch, watching the rain, feeling the heat of the day swept away beneath ferocious clouds. My hand rests on my heart near my throat, feeling the slender, fragile bones in my neck stand out as I turn my head to watch hummingbirds zip between raindrops.

I have often wondered how other people do it, how they write real books. Now, I wonder how I, myself am doing it. I don't know how, I think, but I am doing it anyway. Then, heart beating beneath thin skin, raindrops spinning through the air, breathing in the wild thunder-stained air, I do know. Breath by breath. Step by step. Word by word. Page by page. Poem by poem.

Yoga on Mount Doom

I dreamed I practiced yoga
at the Gates of Mordor
rolling my purple mat
out carefully on parched
and barren ground.
Balancing on one leg
I extended my hand across
a fiery and forbidden horizon,
leg arching backward
into dancer's pose,
the quintessential
pose of destination yogis.
Finding my center
even while
facing
Mount Doom.

The sky is darkening, the sun patched over with gathering clouds. The deck is littered with leaves, some holding perfect raindrops cupped along their veins. The sky is blue in the east, dotted with rolls of white clouds. In the west, there are gray shadows pressing on the sky. A bundle of leaves drops suddenly from the treetops, making its way with sequential crashes from branch to branch, like some sort of ominous advancing creature in a movie.

I begin my pacing circuits around the deck and see Mark in the front yard starting to burn trash. We burn our household paper trash a few times a year on a wet day after a good rain. The smoke billows from the burn barrel around to the back deck, enveloping me in a drifting fog that dissipates into the trees as I step, foot by careful foot, along the planks.

How can I get myself back? I wonder. It feels like the only answer is to get even smaller and to do *even less*. To watch the world spin on without me as I curl into a destiny as small—and as infinite—as a twenty-foot expanse of gray boards. I am no longer arrogant enough to think I can tell anyone else how to do it. I am not certain enough to claim any answers and I don't feel smart enough to lay out any roadmaps, encouragement, or how tos for anyone else.

I notice small particles of ash drifting in front of me and my mind turns to my past students, when I taught college classes in human services, and something I used to tell them: *We have to be careful that we are not teaching our clients how to live in hell and like it.*

When I would say this, I was referring to guarding against teaching our clients techniques and skills for adapting to, conforming to, or acquiescing to oppressive systems. When we consider people in the context of their environment and the things they need to be healthy and thriving, often it is the environment which needs to make changes, not the person. It has been said that "it is no measure of health to be well-adapted to a profoundly sick society." I wonder about my own life stage: *am I adapting with grace and openness to the circumstances in which I find myself, or am I adapting to powerlessness and restriction?*

The Underworld, as Persephone knows it, is not the same as "hell" as in the Christian conception as a punishment of eternal torment. The Underworld in Greek myth is a shadowy realm beneath the earth which may be a place for lost souls, a waystation for travelers on their journey to the next realm. Persephone hears the cries of lost souls and is there to guard and guide their passage through the Underworld realms. However, much as I do not wish to teach myself to live in hell and like it, I do not want to resign myself to a shadowed Underworld existence either. I am willing to undertake a journey seeking my soul, but I want to return, rebuilt, renewed, and restored.

Turn and Face Yourself

May you make space
to turn and face yourself.

This is my message from morning, drifting into my mind with the first moments of a new day.

The sky is clear, the sun is bright between the trees. The tufted titmice creak and buzz, while the bugs are mysteriously silent. Two blue jays dip overhead, changing course in midair as they see me standing on the deck, checkered tails illuminated in the sunshine. A spider web floats lazily between oaks, the spider in the center swaying gently, lit from behind. A second spider web, larger, drifts into view, stair-stepped behind the first. The wind picks up briefly and the webs ripple, tethered skillfully in place, but flexible enough to sway with changes.

Behind them, low in the woods, the first hawk's call rises.

What would it take to face myself? I wonder. I begin to imagine long days of solitude, alone with books, journals, time, silence, and prayers, to really dig in, to stare into my own eyes, to discover what is there and what I know. But, then I realize with a jolt, facing myself means not just in silence with colored pens and a cup of tea in the rose petals as the sun rises, but also under raindrops, in home physical therapy, in making dinner, in listening to friends, in hitting print on the shipping labels, and in scooping a small boy on roller skates off the floor where he has fallen.

If I think I am only "real" or whole in moments of solitude and personal reflection, I will spend a lot of time starving for myself. If I can face myself in each moment, hold my center, stay connected within other action, be alert for the magic of place and the mystery of the everyday even while typing or talking or reading Harry Potter to my kids, then every day is an intense and endlessly amazing laboratory for growth, discovery, and change.

What if I accepted myself as whole, real, and true wherever I go, bringing myself back in, with just a single conscious breath of awareness, with open eyes, with a moment to place a hand on my heart and know without a doubt... This. Is. It.?

I look up just in time to see a beautiful crow crest the top of the roof and fly above me. Moments later, a second crow swoops above the roof, low enough that I can distinguish separate black feathers in its wing. It spots me with a black eye, pulling up somewhat comically in midair and adjusting its flight path so it crosses over the mulberry tree instead of my head.

I finish reading *The Long Journey Home,* an anthology of writing about Demeter and Persephone edited by Christine Downing. Much of it is from a Jungian, psychoanalytic perspective, which isn't a match for much of my own understanding of myth, psychology, and spirituality, but the book contains other seeds of wisdom and understanding as well. In an essay by Laura Sims, she writes: *If this is being lost, then I have found my way. It is not necessary to remember who we are. One can't take oneself too seriously.*

It is a needed reminder... I can't think my way out of this. I can't solve myself as a problem. I can't force myself to move faster or to learn more quickly. I have to continue looking, listening, and feeling my way through.

Stitches Back in Time

My daughter is leaving for a week at camp. The blanket on her bed that she also wants to take with her is a blue quilt my grandma made for me in 1984, when I was five. This quilt was on my bed for most of my childhood and went to my dorm room bed with me, and then onto the bed in my first apartment.

After I got married and no longer had a twin bed, it was folded into the blanket box, emerging only when someone needed an extra blanket, to cover kids at sleepovers, and so forth until it made its way onto my daughter's bed when she moved into her own room. My older sons have quilts on their beds that my grandma made for them, but she died when my daughter was two and so Alaina uses this one, the same quilt that wrapped my own girlhood. When I fold it up to pack for her today, my hand catches on my grandma's initials, carefully stitched there thirty-five years ago and yet still, at work in the world.

I read a quote in Natalie Goldberg's book *Writing Down the Bones* about how reading a poem written 150 years ago brings that poet's breath back into being as you speak their words. I feel like these stitches bring my grandmother's hands back into being. She wasn't a particularly physically demonstrative person, but she demonstrated her love for us in other, tangible ways and we still quite literally carry something of her touch in our days.

A memory comes back to me, one of those childhood moments that stands out vividly as important. I am sitting with my grandmother at the kitchen table. In passing, she pinches the skin on the back of her hand and shows me how it takes moment to sink back down, remaining for a fractional time as a tiny standing ridge of flesh. She tells me that she remembers seeing the skin on her own grandmother's hands do that too and it surprises her to see it in her own hands, that when she passes the mirror she still expects to see a girl there, but instead there is an old woman. I later inherited one of her rings, the one shaped like a golden ball that I used to love to twist around her finger as I sat on her lap as a child. It fits on the same finger on my hand that it fit on hers. Someday, I wonder, will I show my own future granddaughter a pinched piece of skin on my own hand.

The grandmother whose hands she speaks of, my great-great grandmother Caroline, drew beautiful little sketches of small landscapes and household items. One of her drawings, of a small seaside tower, hangs in my own living room, next to a quilt pieced by my grandmother, Lyla, and a felted picture created by my mother, Barbara. All these works of our hands, the motherline, one creative woman birthing the next.

For now, my mother shows my daughter how to crochet and knits me wool socks to wear. Our kitchen cupboards are filled with her pottery. I make goddesses for a living and spin poems from spider webs and stones. It is in making things for and with one another that the mothers and daughters in my family most consistently share our love. It is right here, made visible on feet and bed and wall and page.

I come from a long line of makers and doers. After my grandmother dies and I am going through clippings and memorabilia for her memorial service, which I am honored to priestess for our family, I learn that she once organized a women's conference titled: "Stop the world, we want to get on." And now, here I am, hungering too to "stop the world," only this time it is because I need to step off for a moment, to pause.

There is Nothing Tidy Here

Outside, the boards are slick and dark with rain. The sky is gray and a brisk wind stirs up and fades and whirls again. Thin fingers of mist rise up from the valley and the deck is strewn with small, yellow leaves. I can feel another change in the air already. We have just settled into the bite and berries of summer and yet autumn now whispers just around the corner. A year is both very long and very short all at once. I hear a squawk as I begin my circles and just see a black crow above the roof, dipping back into the trees of the west.

I am unsure what I am seeking any longer: *is it time, the self, Goddess, connection, magic? Is it just awareness and as much ease and joy as can bloom in the margins? Is it a radical restructuring of life, business, relationship, and family? Or is it an opportunity to consciously rebuild my soul, each moment an opportunity for mindfulness, for awareness, for pausing to really breathe in the reality of it all?*

In *Simple Abundance* Sarah Ban Breathnach quotes Evelyn Underhill, an early twentieth century mystic and writer as believing:

Women mystics with worldly responsibilities often became visionaries, prophetesses because they were able to combine "spiritual transcendence with great practical ability." Be they poets, saints, or cooks, they "remained all their lives the devout lovers of reality while seeking Spirit."

As I reflect on these words, the phrase: *There is nothing tidy here,* rings through my head like a mantra, like a moral, like a conclusion.

Tiny raindrops begin to mist my writing and I step out onto the deck again, feeling the rain. I circle several times as it builds from a misting to full, cool drops and then I duck back under the cover of the roof, stepping mindfully along the covered side porches to finish my half mile, singing. The song winds through raindrops like a healing salve, a rallying cry, a declaration of wholeness. Once Persephone is honored with three rounds of the prayersong my half mile is complete, wind- and rain-accompanied and hope-laced. I stand at the edge of the covered part of the deck and open my arms in my morning blessing and then bring my hands to my belly, heart, and forehead for my three breaths.

As I open my eyes again, I know. It truly is at least a year I need to spend with Persephone. I'm still getting going, I'm still scratching the surface of what it could mean to journey with her, to walk with her, to learn from her, to explore her stories, symbols, and myths. I wanted it to be tidy, neatly organized, but there is nothing tidy here. This is an unraveling, a reweaving, an unraveling again, step by sometimes limping step through an Underworld of change and evolving lessons. I am writing myself back into being and I am learning that when I am alert each day to the story of my life, there is continuity and power, an unfolding discovery. The crow from this morning is not separated from the three crows of three months ago, they each contribute a step on the journey. Writing each morning, observing each morning, is teaching me how all these steps fit together. Tidy, no. Whole, yes.

As I stand, looking into the rain, a hummingbird whirrs into view, hovering amongst the still green poke berries and remaining white flowers, before zipping away between raindrops.

Limpy

I dream of hiking in the Smoky Mountains, a winding trail laid round green peaks. A woven triangle of sticks sits in the middle of the path.

I walk through a spider web strung through the mulberry tree, singing. I am preoccupied and distracted. The clock is ticking on the workday beginning. I try to appreciate the cool air, looking up to see a waning half-moon tilted in the clear blue sky.

I think: *there are beginnings and there are endings. Don't like one so much that you forget the other, or neglect the middle, where all the juice of living resides.*

It is radical to witness this morning and dare to tell about it: sun shining through the walnut tree, rooster crowing from a nearby neighbor's home, bird-song lilting over cricket song through cool, sweet air.

Even though I don't "have time," I sit in the chair, feeling the sun soak into my eyelids, listening to the hummingbirds battle above the elderberries and to the unseen cardinal singing merrily in front of me. It quickly grows hot under the direct sun, but as I offer my breaths to Persephone, a cool breeze snakes in from the west to curl delicately up my neck and around my arm.

I am open to your guidance.

I am open to what is.

We don't finish working until seven in the evening. I feel tight and constrained, eager for change and some sense of balance. The air is cool and inviting. It has been six weeks since my fall, and we decide to walk on the gravel road. My proprioception is back, I can once more perceive my ankle and foot in time and space and unconsciously adjust to the variations in the uneven terrain. I feel exhilarated to be free again, to be on the road, to see something new.

Rising from the withered and crunchy remains of June's flowers, poison ivy, and the remaining blackberries, the tall, straight, proud bursts of sawtooth sunflowers. I am thrilled to be seeing them, thrilled to be here, thrilled to be back on the road. We hear a rustling and spy a gray armadillo, riffling through the brown leaves beneath the trees. I pause and point, peering at its prehistoric form rummaging in the leaf cover.

We decide to turn back after a mile, I am limping a little again now, but my heart feels full and happy, holding hands with Mark, walking down the road together. I have so missed doing this.

As we pass the neighbor's house, we spot a doe in the field with her two fawns. She sees us and starts to run away. We are surprised to see that she is Limpy, the lame doe that we have seen in the area for the last three years, somehow making her life work despite the fact that her poorly healed leg points in the wrong direction. I feel there is a message in here somewhere for me, seeing this wounded but still walking mother with her twin babies, both of us knowing what it is like to stand our painful ground in a green field under the broad, blue sky.

> *There is magic to be found*
> *in an untidy life*
> *in an untidy world*
> *where nothing stays the same*
> *and growth*
> *is always possible.*

Disappointments

My ankle feels achy and tight this morning and I look forward to the day when I no longer notice it. However, there is also something to be said for, and learn from, deliberate movement, careful steps, considered action, conscious momentum.

I feel distant and distracted, my mind moving through the to-dos of the day, the workshop I am supposed to teach this afternoon, the shower I need to take, the picnic I need to pack. I have to consciously, deliberately pause my circles and tip my head to the blue sky, the half-moon hanging above the roof, tilted and solemn. I hear a few high, distant hawk calls and then silence.

The air is cool and welcome again and I finish my half-mile sojourn before I realize I haven't sung. My mind is elsewhere, not on these deliberate steps around gray boards as morning settles onto dew-wet blackberry leaves and globes of still-green pokeberries, illuminated from behind as they curve over sun-warped railings to sway delicately over the planks of wood.

I do sing then. I pray. I open my arms to the sky. I offer my breaths. It is all that I have today.

Inside I realize I am out of time for yoga and feel the tight sensation of being "sped up" within my chest, choosing between self-care—self-maintenance, really—and commitment to other tasks of living. I think of friends I have seen over the summer, planning events, rushing from place to place, obligation to obligation. From my current position, wounded on the sidelines, I've found myself thinking more and more often as I watch them and think of my own life of scurrying:

It doesn't have to be this way. You have a choice. Life can be different. It is possible to feel ease instead of rushing.

I know this to be true. I've felt it with increasing frequency over the last months. There is a difference between feeling at home in your life, stable in your soul, and being fractured by many demands. It takes courage, commitment, and devotion to continue to defend your edges, to protect your margins, to rebuild your soul, to hold your center, to breathe peace. It is an ongoing process of remembering, of renegotiating, of yielding, and of holding your ground.

My card from the *Sacred Traveler Oracle* today is Solitude and my Woman-rune is the Circle, rune of the self. My rune yesterday was the Cauldron. *Am I listening?* I hunger, still, for time to steep.

May you thrive.
May you know your own power.
May you sit with peace
and walk with patience.

The homeschool workshop is poorly attended and by the time we reach my own afternoon session there are six people total participating, three of them are leading sessions, which leaves three people to split between us. No one chooses my session, carefully prepared over three days, and I decide I will leave early.

I feel a sense of eager anticipation approaching the lake at the park across the road. This is where I really met Persephone for the first time, felt her words twining on the wind and out my fingertips. The grass and clover are littered with goose poop and some actual litter as well. I hear the watery warble of a red-winged blackbird right away and feel my heart lift. Tanner is with me and we find a white and gray dove's feather and then goose and duck feathers as well, skirting copious poop as we exclaim together over our finds. A dove soars over my head and a blackbird settles on the ferny-looking branches of a cypress tree. I look up into its branches, broad and green and glowing in the vibrancy of summer, and see it is laden with green cones, dipping the tips of the branches towards the earth.

Two men in a small orange cart drive by along the edges of the baseball diamond in the park and I notice they are spraying poison along the edges of the fence surrounding the baseball field and around the pitcher's mound. The wind shifts and some of the spray blows towards us. I feel the taste in the back of my throat and my sense of water's edge reverie and learning is abruptly halted. I turn away from them and gaze out into the expanse of water, wishing there was no poison being poured onto the ground behind me, but still feeling a palpable sense of stillness and solace here in this place. Two empty Fireball Whiskey bottles lie tilted at the bottom of a cypress, the roots which knot into abstract art at the edge of the lake, puffy white clouds reflected in the still, grey-green water.

Tanner steps in a mass of slimy green poop and my reflections end. I pick my way back to the car with him noticing two vultures circling around the park and only later realizing I didn't sing or make my offering to Persephone here, at her lake between the worlds. This is a portal place, I can feel it, between earth and sky.

Take a breath
at the edge of desire and choice...
What do you truly want?
What does your heart whisper?
Are you listening?
Is there enough space for you
in your own life?

I'm not sure if there is, but I do know what it feels like, tastes like...

Bumping along the gravel road back home, I think about never going to a group function of any kind at all, fantasizing about a life of monastic, spiritual devotion to the Goddess from my hilltop home. I am headachy and irritable after my long day in town for not much benefit. I feel cross and short-tempered about having wasted my time and caught up in thoughts about what we are doing over the next three days. *Why do I continue to feel so hampered in my choice-making, bound by constraints of my own making or of other people's possibly imaginary expectations or wishes of me?*

My insight about it not having to be this way lingers in my mind, dancing, whispering, full of potential and promise.

It doesn't have to be this way. You can choose.

In the studio, looking through the walls Mark is framing out into the wide field beyond, overgrown with all manner of botanical mysteries and delights, I spot a single coneflower, low and sweet, right by the wall. And then, inside as I defrost food for dinner, report to my kids about my "failed" workshop and munch on leftover cookies, I see a bright flare of red outside the kitchen window. It is one of the blazing penstemon flowers that we planted last year, escaped from the flower box and growing rouge amid the iris bulbs. I love seeing it, bright and free, thriving in a place it has chosen for itself.

Tender Breast

As I circle the deck this morning, I think of outrage culture, so much experience and life compressed into tiny memes often designed to provoke and antagonize. I feel awash with sadness about climate change and the health of the earth, reading articles that say we have only eighteen months left to take significant action before permanent catastrophic change is locked into motion. I worry that we are causing this very thing through our own hopelessness, pessimism and negative predictions. But, we are also causing it through corporate culture and convenience and an inability to really look. I feel defeated and uneasy, but the air is cool and the birds sing and the trees glow and right here, all around me, are signs of abundant growth and vibrant, determined, irrepressible life. The earth is not dying. Humanity is changing and humans themselves are at risk. We cannot be seduced into despair by fear. We must live out loud, with our arms open to the moon, the sun, the rain, and the whirling wonder of it all.

I consciously extract fear from my brain and sing the Persephone prayersong. My mind clears and my heart lifts as I step and sing. I remember what I used to tell my college students:

It requires no courage to be seduced into cynicism, to capitulate to a plodding dullness of spirit that refuses to believe in change.

I am feeling a pain and tightness either in my actual breast or in my chest wall and as I lie down on the boards, body fully extended, for my three breaths, I think: *do not store anger in your tender breast.*

Am I storing anger here? I think so, though I'm not exactly sure what about or where it wants to go.

I need this time to settle into myself. I think about homeschool co-op, the tug on my energy, reserves and resources. *It doesn't have to be like this. You do have a choice.* I know the difference between feeling good, happy, and balanced and not. *How do I guard that? Protect myself? Take action to preserve my own delicate, passionate, powerful spirit?*

After my breaths, I think of Noah, our third baby, who died in my second trimester. I remember how fresh the grief was, how raw and uncertain and ruinous of my identity, my trust, my faith, my living. I think of how it has faded away now, become invisible, no longer split open and wounded, no longer sharp, but that, ten years later, our family still holds a place for him. Moments from my pregnancy flood into me for a few minutes, as clear as chapters of a story, necessary to the unfolding.

I take another breath and rise up into a seated position once more, gazing into the creaking, groaning, bleeding, singing, breathing, wild world.

Do not store anger
in your tender breast,
the soft territory
of your humanity
requires room to roam.
Let yourself range through
landscapes of pain and joy
until you weave together
a cloak of power.
Let buried grief rise up
and spill over onto
sunstreaked ground.
Breathe in and know
you are whole.
Breathe out and know
you are here.
Sit with everything
until you know
what you need to do.
The answers are there,
waiting beneath
your thin and magic
skin.

The Element of Earth

I wake with breast pain again, or is it chest pain? I can't tell which it is.

The moon is a thinning silver crescent in the blue sky, the clouds form a puffy palm around it, stubby fingers extended with the moon cradled between two of them, creased and seamed like a real hand. A black and yellow swallowtail butterfly coasts along the gentle air surrounding me and the sound of neighboring chickens rises with the cicadas into the air.

I have brought my new *Herbcrafter's Tarot* by Joanna Colbert and Latisha Guthrie with me this morning. I love how the cards are reflected in my actual environment. I have decided to photograph the ones I can along with their living counterparts in my own yard. I take a picture with mint, with raspberry, and with elderberry, again feeling enchanted and grateful to have access to these allies right outside my own doors. I take pictures of a translucent sunrise goddess in the light filtering behind pokeberries, green against their beautiful red-purple stalks. Puffs of wild lettuce seed are illuminated behind them. Poke is poisonous to humans, but nourishing and valuable to birds. Wild lettuce is hallucinogenic to humans, I'm not sure about birds, but it makes me remember that there is very little that is black and white about the world, life, being here, now.

This is my work with Earth as it has been evolving since Summer Solstice. The wildflowers, the morning glories, the many lessons from the roadside ecosystem, the deer, the snakes, the turtles, the butterflies, the crows, all are communicators, teachers, and sharers from the element of Earth. I am moving through these layers of initiation with the elements that I have sensed at work with me since spring.

In the evening, as the bread bakes for dinner, we set off for just one mile on the gravel road. At the end of the driveway, we look down the road to see Limpy and one baby as well as another larger deer. The tightness of a long day at the computer and putting labels on envelopes fades as soon as we see the sky and feel the air. I run through a litany of seeds I hope to harvest before the summer is over: vervain, milkweed (both pink and white), evening primrose, butterfly flower, indigo, blazing star, and rosehips from the pink prairie roses that twine low along the roadside. I imagine the sides of our driveway and the berm outside the new studio alive with color and life.

The mullein is about to bloom, the first yellow flowers opening on the tall, straight lances of fuzzy leaves, reaching to the heavens. The bright sawtooth sunflowers make us smile and as we lean over to look at them, a great cacophony of crow sound rises from the woods right by us, raucous, loud, disturbed. We see several crows swoop and dive away from the trees, more caws rising from the roadside, and then they all drift away, yelling and calling as they resettle deeper in the woods. Standing on the road, looking off into the enchanted acres, I can't help but feel somehow barred from a magical land by the roadside barriers of summer: thorn, poison ivy, and thick, rambunctious growth. It is as if I can feel the magic pulsing, leaking over, tantalizing me with a small glimpse via the black wings of these crows.

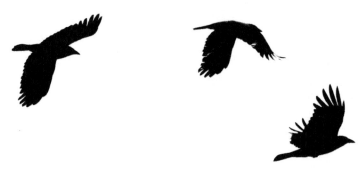

Anniversary

It is our twenty-first wedding anniversary. We are unsure what to do to celebrate, picking through options that all feel stale and hollow. Our brains feel incapable of making a decision. What we truly want—a day home alone together without kids or employees—is impossible. Everything else feels forced or just not fun. We do know that we don't want to spend it working.

We go for a walk around the lake at the park where Mark first asked me out twenty-four years ago. That day, we'd been teaching Boy Scouts how to make rope in the park for six hours. Something in both of our teenage hearts knew that we were fundamentally compatible, but I marvel that they also sensed we'd still be able to make things together every day, two decades later. The tension I've been carrying inside me relaxes at last, and I finally feel present in this day, clicking in to now, this moment, instead of feeling tethered by the bonds of the undone.

We stop on the bridge where he asked me out and take a selfie, my hair blowing in the wind, our bodies feeling warm and easy with satisfaction as we smile into my phone. We make a complete circuit around the lake. My steps are almost normal, though I feel a constant small ache in my ankle that lets me know I still need to pay careful attention, but I am so very grateful to be here, doing this.

Mark mentions that this anniversary marks the point at which he's spent as many years married to me as he spent not married to me and I reach out to hold his hand. As I look at him, time suddenly collapses and I see those young people and everything they didn't know they would experience together and I also see forward, into our future, and all the things we still don't yet know: the hard things we will have to do together as we age, as our kids leave us, as our health declines, the journey we still have to take with each other.

Remember how we thought it would all be easy, I say, and my eyes fill with tears.

We were right, he says.

We have done lots of hard things together, things we couldn't have imagined back then, but being married to you has always been soft and easy.

I can't keep talking, there are tears collecting in my eyes and trickling down my face. Marriage has been soft, gentle, warm, and easy for us: a safe place to be full and whole, held and known. I think of holding him at his father's graveside twenty years ago; of the death of our third baby; of him wiping blood off my legs after I gave birth and now patiently rubbing my sore ankle every morning and every night. Life has definitely been harder than we knew it could be sometimes and we have had bumps in our road—pain, grief, stress, and struggle—but we've always been on the same "team," always looking the same direction, facing whatever difficulty.

Later, we head to the river, admiring the coneflowers and tall bellflowers waving along the roadside. It feels important to me to fully immerse in the spring water. I have only stepped in it twice this year. I haven't even been to the river land since the week I was hurt. Today I successfully, but slowly, navigate the steep path down to the water and then wade down to the quadruple confluence, where our two small spring-fed creeks that originate on the land, a wet-weather creek that runs through, and the river that curves in from the west, meet and become one. I slide down the rocks into the confluence and after some moments of hesitation in the freezing water, I immerse myself up to my neck. I am seeking the sensation of cleansing and rebirth I have felt here before, the lifting of everything else and the feeling of emerging renewed.

Dragonflies dance over the water. Small fish dip and swirl around me, nibbling at the skin of my ankles and feet and then, as I lie back to float in the water, at my thighs and bottom as well. The river birch trees are tall, leaning over the water from their tenuous, land-sustaining hold on the river-bank, their roots forming the boundaries of this waterway. The sunlight catches in their papery, curling bark, making them glow, and I wonder, briefly, at how much time, chance, and opportunity has gone into their becoming trees here, now, after being one of a million seeds, seeking purchase and opportunity near watery, but difficult ground.

We sit in the cold river confluence, talking and looking at the trees. It feels so good to be here, alone in our marriage without our kids, remembering who we are together, unbound and free in newborn water.

Cauldron Month

I dream of a mossy pool in which a gigantic turtle-like creature rests, shell covered with thick, waving mosses. My feet are in the water and it swims over to me, nearly invisible against the thick, green bottom of the pool, and nudges my feet, tipping to one side so the soles of my feet pass over the moss of its back.

My mind turns to Cauldron Month in August. I haven't done many preparations for it and yet, I desperately need it.

I have honored a Cauldron Month for myself for the last three years and it is always a very powerful time. Each year, I crave the opportunity to do it again. August as a Cauldron Month means a time in which I "take it all to the cauldron" and let it bubble and brew and stew and percolate. This means that while our shop will be open for most of the month and orders will be processed like usual, I am pulling my energy further inward to let myself listen and be and to see what wants to emerge. I take time to reflect:

What am I cooking?
What flavors do I want to add?
What do I want to create?

What needs time and focus to bubble and brew?
Can I allow myself to steep in my own flavors?

I sit down to write some notes about all the things I'd like to stop doing or pull back from as I steep, noticing that I've really been trying to do this all year, with varying success, as "life always rushes in to fill the void," to paraphrase Anne Morrow Lindberg. Suddenly the shadow of wings passes over me and I almost jump, looking up to see a vulture coasting by. I feel startled back into reality, back where I want and need to be. *Thank you,* I call, *I love you!*

In Jennifer Louden's book *Comfort Secrets for Busy Women,* she writes about choice and the process of choosing:

> *The woman who knows when to use her will and when to put it away creates the life she is meant to have... It is basic yet so hard to verbalize because it is in the void that we must wait. When we get overly fixated on doing or caring for others to prove our worth, we cut ourselves off from our mysterious source of being. We have to start in the goalless place and wait there, hushing and holding, until gradually the unfolding of our next step is revealed...opening to what life is bringing and then working with that opening is how we let the inside [of our lives] shape the outside.*

As I think about the day, space and ease, how to structure my days, my Cauldron Month to come in August, our work life. I hear: *let it be as easy as breath.*

> *Let it be as easy as breath.*
> *Let it be as effortless as bone.*
> *Let it be as fluid as tears.*
> *Let it be as harmonious as a heartbeat.*
> *Let it be as silent as the dance of neurons*
> *through space.*
> *Let it be as unconscious as dreaming.*
> *Let it be as slow as,*
> *as soft as,*
> *as whole as,*
> *as smooth as,*
> *you are.*
> *Let all be easy in your temple,*
> *and listen to the singing in your skin.*

Seeds of Anticipation

I am in the front yard, seeking plantain. I'm working through the *Herbcrafter's Tarot* day by day and the Aces are all tall, spear-like plants, reaching for the sky. The plantain in the yard is tired, leaves peppered with holes, but the long lances of seeds bob and wave and wait for me. I've been planning to make a goddess grid for Lammas and after kneeling by the plantain, I start to cast my eyes around for other likely mandala materials. At first I don't find anything, everything seems dry, thirsty, wilted, parched, gone to seed. But then I start to recognize the seeds and to be excited by the connections to the themes of the holiday. I pick small pink flower-seed heads from a plant I can't name, I pick plantain seeds and amaranth seeds and wild rye and ironweed blooms and small spikes of yellow flowers. A single dandelion, a single Queen Anne's Lace bloom, and eight blackberries join the growing collection tucked in the makeshift basket of my shirt. I feel awash with gratitude that these things are all *here*, waiting for me, or not waiting for me, just being here, together.

A skink with a partially regrown tail catches my eye as it crawls down the outer wall of the house, a cardinal flies into the trees, and a black and white dragonfly hovers overhead.

As I carry everything back to the deck to arrange on my grid board, I feel settled and calm, easy and connected. However, I also find myself wondering as I think about what a good picture this will make: *how much is for social media consumption and how much is from within? How much is an interweaving of the two?* I want to create magic and meaning for myself. If it can reach out and touch the lives of others so much the better, but I need to guard against creating *only* for the audience, for the likes, for the comments.

As I look at the items nestled in my shirt, I see a flaky seed from one of the grass stems, it looks like one of the river oats, but it walks. It is actually an insect, perfectly shaped and colored to match the seeds of the stems on which it travels.

I build my grid and it is exciting to discover how well the pieces work together: the amaranth curling into the rye, the blackberries making a flower in the center. They connect to the themes and intentions of Lammas so well: the harvest, our gratitude. I feel fortunate to live in a place where our weather and wild growth so tidily and neatly mirrors the "traditional" turn of the wheel, the experiences of the eight seasonal holidays. As I work, a tiny puff of another seed drifts through the air in front of me, glowing in the morning sunbeams, and lands on the boards. I think of how to connect with the magic of place and it floods into me how I would share it with others: *look for things that grow, look for things that move, look for things for that fly.*

I put my hands on either side of the finished grid, breathing in and out with appreciation, gratitude, respect, and pleasure. I feel in the presence of magic, here, with these seeds and flowers and sunshine.

After I lie back for my breaths, I rise to see that the sun has moved. The grid is dappled with shadows from the mulberry tree, and the single dandelion flower is illuminated and glowing, in its place of honor at the Lammas moon.

AUGUST

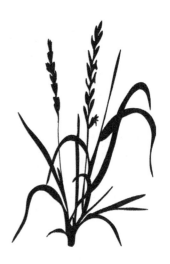

Lammas

I wake early, glowing with alertness, humming with glee, alive in all my senses, and full to bursting with possibility. I feel full of exhilaration, a sort of irrepressible, bubbling excitement and anticipation. This is the magic of the Cauldron: the first tendrils of steam beginning to rise, the blending of new flavors bubbling. I recognize something in me trying to wrestle with or control the sensation, tamp it down, rein it in, argue with it, so I consciously let the bubbling joy wash through me completely, as I have let waves of less positive emotion and thought fill me over the last several months of this process. There is a wild excitement here, an anticipatory flood of something fresh and stimulating.

> *Between the shadow*
> *and the shine*
> *there is a place that*
> *needs your time.*

These words ring through my head as I brush my teeth and prepare for the day.

It is dark at first outside, but then an orange glow begins to light the room and as I sit on the floor writing, I hear a hawk call briefly outside the bedroom window.

I feel untethered.

As I step outside, another Cauldron prayer begins to swirl from within me and I write before I walk, circling a few times and adding new lines as I make my rounds.

Guide me into the depths
where I might steep in my own knowing
and discover questions
I've forgotten how to ask.
Let me brew into complexity,
richness,
and depth,
as I drink deeply from
my own life
and savor the flavor
in this cauldron of being,
becoming,
birthing,
and breathing.

In the evening we prepare for a very simple family Lammas ritual. I don't feel inspired to do anything elaborate, so we cut our loaf of special bread, prepared earlier by my sister-in-law and delivered warm. We add blackberry jelly to our slices and leave one slice for our offering. We step out together onto the deck and set the bread, a candle, and a garnet-colored meditation goddess onto the center of the deck. We speak aloud of our gratitude for the changes, blessings, and creations of the last few weeks and of the months since Imbolc. Then, we each tear off a piece of bread from the extra piece and speak aloud what we will be sacrificing, what we are willing to change in the new season. A pattern emerges from our words, that of a family-wide wish for a better and healthier schedule, earlier dinner-times and bed-times, more opportunities to play together. We join hands and close our micro-ritual with our favorite blessing:

May goddess bless and keep us, may wisdom dwell within us, may we create peace.

—Carol P. Christ

I feel warm and satisfied with this tiny ritual, this simple observance of the season, this connection between the elements to those I love best.

Patterns

The faint sound of the hawks calling greets me in the morning. The air is cool and sweet outside. There are six ragged red roses valiantly blooming on the rosebush by the deck. The ironweed is almost finished, the purple puffs losing their petals, the eyes of the flowers becoming seed. The sky is studded with white clouds in a stuttering, segmented swath across the bowl of blue. I circle for a half-mile, drinking my tea, and thinking of assembling materials for the autumn magic I can taste in the air. I recognize a sensation of staleness with my routine and decide to walk in the driveway instead.

I step along the gravel singing my Persephone prayersong, thin and sweet in the morning air. I am conscious of, and thankful for, the ability of my feet to successfully read and navigate the rocky uneven terrain again. How I took that skillful reading of the land beneath my feet for granted until these last two months of my life.

I think about how each year for the last four years, preceding my Cauldron Time in August, I've been sick and I realize that the ankle injury has continued the pattern for me into this year too. Each year something has happened to me in the summer that has forced me into the Cauldron, even if I was intentionally planning for time spent there.

This year, I didn't see it coming so soon in June, falling down while standing still on my own front porch and doing myself so much damage that here, at the midpoint between summer and fall, I still have pain that radiates from ankle through calf at the end of each day.

With my notifications and apps shut off on my phone in honor of Cauldron Time, I notice unfamiliar spaces in my brain, spaces usually occupied by other people's ideas, opinions, experiences, and needs. I keep rolling my thoughts around the space, like probing an empty tooth socket, noticing that something that was there, is no longer there. Unlike an empty tooth socket, this space feels good. Empty in the best of ways. Inviting.

My mind turns again to choice and force. *Why do I continue to fear that unless I force myself, I won't do something that matters or is important?* Tanner comes to ask me to excavate one of my doll accessory sets from the bowels of the closet for him. I tell him that that isn't going to be something I do today. He wheedles and begs, pressuring me to do it and I tell him that I feel like he is trying to force me and I'm not going to be doing things by force today.

I wonder if it could possibly be this simple: *if it feels like force, don't do it.* It is okay to let desire and ease be your guides. You can trust yourself. You've never given yourself any reason to doubt that you can.

I make my collage goddess with a background of yellow sunflowers and a blue temple door in her center. I put transparent feathers across her head, heart, and base. I cut the remainder of the blueberry, gooseberry, and raspberry stickers apart and gather them into a bunch at one hip, by the door. I combine words from two recent poems into her message: *there is nothing tidy here. Let the wildflowers of the roadsides teach you what it means to live.* She feels happy and settled, at peace with her place.

New Moon at Dusk

We walk on the road at dusk. The crows have already gone to bed, but a lone deer watches us carefully from across the field. The white moonflowers are still tight closed trumpets under the sliver of the new moon. A small brave bunny meets our eyes with its black ones, quivering slightly as we greet it, but holding its ground, nose twitching, head dipping down for another nip of sweet grass. We find a perfect blue butterfly dead in the road, wings whole and unblemished.

We talk about community building, about nourishing friendships, me musing at my extinguished steam for holding groups together. Mark mentions that he's never had this and wonders aloud whether one of the reasons I no longer feel I do is because I work nearly full time on our business now, the first time I've worked full time since 2000.

I recall the audiobook I have been listening to, *Burnout.* The authors, Amelia

Nagoski and Emily Nagoski speak of "Human Giver Syndrome" and describe how women are punished for opting out of this damaging, but intensely socially reinforced, pattern of expected behavior. They also note that we, heavily socialized into this model, may try to unconsciously punish others when we see or sense that they are opting out of the model. *Yes,* I say, *most of the relational work of the world is built and sustained by the unpaid emotional labor of women.*

I had forgotten about how I felt like I owed people my time, my energy, my resources, how I offered myself up to be consumed to demonstrate my own worthiness. At this point in my life, I don't miss it, but at some point, I can see wishing to rebuild the fabric of community connection too. Right now, though, it is all the parts of my soul that I gave away, starved, or malnourished in an effort to be worthy and loved that I recall to me, that I rebuild in me, that I wish to feed with my time and my tenderness.

Freedom of Joy

The hawk calls at dawn, high, shrill, and insistent, a summoning. The air is beautifully cool, cold almost, and I snuggle and doze for another hour before rising. When I do get up, the hawk is still. The bugs too are quiet, the sun glowing behind the dead oak tree. Some of the poke berries have ripened to black, shining among their still-green sisters. The elderberries, patient and slow, are still green, a spray of firm, tiny pearls, tall and proud, rising up from the raspberry thicket.

I hear the hawk call twice more, high and distant, barely reaching my ears.

> *Let your own self rush in to fill these empty spaces left*
> *when the noises of others' opinions is silenced*
> *and you are alone in your own head.*

I walk on the gravel road for a half-mile, singing first my sun and bones song and then my Persephone prayersong.

Back on the deck, I am feeling stale and still curious about what's next as well as feeling like I'm missing some kind of magic. The Cauldron is an uncomfortable place sometimes. I know I am seeking a hit of magic today, the thrill and joy of discovery, investigation, learning, and I just don't feel it. I almost sit up and go inside, giving up, but then something nudges me to continue, to stay with this muddiness, this ennui, this frustration with paradox.

I feel the soft air curling around me, I hear the bugs groaning, and a woodpecker's fluting call. I reach out to Persephone and then to Medusa too. *What next? Where do I go now?*

Be *patient.*
Let *yourself settle.*

I do actually always know what to do next on a practical level, I remember. I've always been exquisitely capable of guiding my own behavior, choices, tasks, and work. I don't want to lose that internal drive and self-motivation and the continued inspiration I usually feel, that is a gift. What I want to lose is the compulsion, the unconscious element of the drive that just keeps revving, regardless of my own human limits and the callings of my soul. There is balance to be found between breathing, listening and being and the dynamic, thrilling, alchemy of creation.

> *I offer my breath from my belly, the cauldron of creation.*
> *I offer my breath from my heart, the cauldron of compassion.*
> *I offer my breath from my mind, the cauldron of curiosity.*

Is it truly that I'm trying to "figure it all out" so everything, everything, will then feel easy? So I will never again feel wound up, stressed, strained, and pushed? Maybe that *is* what I think is possible, what I am seeking. When really, some level of occasional stress or strain is simply a part of being human. Is it? *Does life become stale, dull, predictable, and stolid when not spiced with the excitement of change, the thrill of growth, the dynamic tension of pushing yourself to reach and create and build and grow?* The introverted side of me that clamors desperately for time, always more time, and stillness, creeping around my consciousness pleading for attention when I am overwhelmed, now seems to have little to say, want, or do, but feels restless and picky, looking for something to experience or taste in the juice of life. *Do I really want stillness, or is that a carrot I dangle in front of myself or even a stick I use to beat myself with?*
NO!
I recognize this.

This is the once again unfamiliar sense of not having too much to do, the tension on the edge before I can't stand the not knowing or the stillness anymore. I let the floodgates open and it all rushes in to fill me, to consume me, to use me, until I recognize the soul-starved part again, reaching, crying, needing, stoking inspiration in fevered moments and stolen silences.

Am I trying to get small enough to never be stressed or am I trying to create a life that is human-sized, that allows for soul-flourishing, that allows space for delight, for joy, for open hours, for bugsong rising on the wind?

I let a different sensation sweep through me: the sensation of ease, of not having too much to do. I can *choose* what fills this space: it doesn't have to be flooded, overfull, exhausted, exhausting. The breeze picks up, and for a moment I have a strong sensation that my breastbone is hollow, the whole center of me is hollow, and the breath and the air rush completely through me easily, cool, calm and empty.

Make me a hollow bone, I remember from earlier this year.

> *Strip this detritus of overdoing back to the bone,*
> *let the sinews of striving slacken and ease,*
> *the knots of muscle and thought soften and still.*
> *The hurry and force float away*
> *and from there,*
> *breathe easy,*
> *heart open,*
> *self hollowed through.*
> *Choose what is next.*

I feel exhilaration now, a rush of energy at having sat through my own discomfort and my twisting questions, at having felt the hollow freedom without having rushed to fill it with activity.

There has been so much that is unnecessary in how I have moved through the world and in my life.

I can unclench.

I can let it flow through the center, calm, open, clear, conscious, connected. *Persephone, where are you?*

> *In the hollow spaces,*
> *always connected.*

I open my planner worksheet for August that I had hoped to use this weekend. Magically, on the top of the page it says: *root deeply to be truly open.* (Danielle LaPorte.)

I choose my cards for the day and from Womanrunes I receive the Cauldron of Dancing Women, the rune of honor, loyalty, and commitment.

I feel like I am waking up from a long dullness, coming around the other side of a shadowy mountain that has obscured my own truth and my own joy for decades through overgiving, overdoing, and overperforming. I am still waking up.

You do not have to overdo to be loved.

You do not have to perform to be loved.

You do not have to worry that your life will become meaningless or pointless if you soften.

This is not about being lazy, this is about being conscious and considered in your choices of how you are filled.

There are many threads that can be loosened without cutting all that binds you to purpose.

Other people in my family history have sometimes seemed to disparage this inner looking, this time for inward exploration, suggesting or outright stating it is selfish, perhaps even mocking it a bit as unnecessary or needless. I feel this generational legacy within as I breathe alone in the sunlight anyway, still with my own self.

Tendrils of air curl around my toes.

Am I getting somewhere? Is there anywhere to go? Without an inner sense of urgency or compulsion to fuel us, will we be okay?

I look at my goddess sculptures, patiently standing sentinel in the sunbeams and stripes of shadow. I feel a sense of certainty that the original thumbprint of the divine is on and in these and that people can feel it. It lives in them.

I want to soak in the Goddess. I want to feel enlivened by her truth, her reality. I want to walk in a state of enchantment and rapturous, continual connection. I want to feel her alive beneath my skin, wrapped through my heart, and woven wildly through all the patterns of my days.

I want to soak in Her, great streams of awareness and living truth.

You can have…
Space to breathe
Room to think
Freedom of choice
Time for joy.

Inhale. Exhale.

As wrote this, I first accidentally typed "you can have freedom of joy." This I can taste too: *freedom of joy.*

Stay Here as Long as Possible

The clouds are white mountains landscaped through the sky. A quiet gray bird sits watchfully in the treetop. The woods feel alive today and I feel expectant, watchful, alert. I feel observed by hundreds of unseen eyes and that my own senses are too technology-dulled to actually spot them. It is amazing what a simple change such as shutting off the notifications on my phone can do. This simple act changing the fabric and the feel of morning. *Who knew that when there is nothing immediately available to you to look at on your phone, you don't look and you don't really need or miss it, you look out at the world instead?*

I watch my feet on the brown gravel, feeling the normal flexion and extension of my joints. *I am grateful, I am grateful, I am grateful,* beats a steady rhythm in my chest with each conscious footfall. A worn woven basket-like square of armadillo skin rests on the rocks, its sandy yellow hatches strong enough to withstand months of tires.

The yellow flowers on the mullein spires have opened more fully and I stop to try to get a photo, goddess teetering on my fingertips beside the muted yellow stars. I return home singing.

The sky has cleared to a soft blue as I lie on the boards for my breaths. I offer Persephone one from my belly, center of being, one from my heart, center of the soul, and one from my mind, center of consciousness.

I am whole, all is well.

For my yoga practice, I listen to an audio-only morning wake up series on Audible with Peter Walters. In one of his cues he encourages us to find a point of balance between being too comfortable and pushing yourself too hard. *Dancing in the space between effort and ease,* he says.

Yes. This is part of what I'm discerning in my own life and work this year. The space between effort and ease. As we do seated spinal twists to close the practice, he says to kiss our knees as we hug them to our chest. I do, feeling silly, but feel a wave of appreciation for my knees and marvel at how little I have thought to ever kiss them in my life.

As he closes the twenty-minute practice Peter whispers, *stay here as long as possible, thank you, I love you,* and I feel a surprising prickle of tears. *Stay here as long as possible.* That is what I'm trying to do with my life this year.

Ease

May you walk in enchantment.
May you dwell in mystery.
May you move in beauty.
May you inhabit curiosity.
May you occupy wonder.
May you serve magic.

We set out onto the gravel road, our faces quickly slicked with sweat even though it is only eight in the morning. As we walk we say that perhaps our word of the year for next year is "ease." Both of us know we wish to welcome more ease and a sense of exhale in the year to come, instead of so much struggling to keep up. It feels good to be aligned together in this intention and idea. Gnats cluster around our eyes and butterflies dance around our ankles as we persist in reaching our first mile of the day.

At home with shiny faces and heavy limbs, Mark shows me the berries on the small Carolina buckthorn trees by the side of the house and I head to the deck for a few minutes alone as our employees start to arrive for the day. As I hear cars pull up to work, I think about our new studio building and how I look forward to its completion: it sometimes feels that people in our house working simply leaves no space for us to breathe.

Standing in the scant shade of the mulberry, the compressor already on for goddess casting, I draw a goddess with a snake curled around her chest and a body patterned with scales. Sweat trickles down my back in hot rivulets like blood. I circle and sing for the last quarter mile of two miles, my leg creaking as I move.

We finish the workday early, all orders completely caught up for the first time in three months. *Is this ease? It is possible?* I am on Lavender, Four of Air, in the *Herbcrafter's Tarot.* It reminds me: *take a break from gathering thoughts and ideas. You have already learned so much. Allow what you have studied to sink into your bones.*

After writing for a few minutes, my mom arrives to carpool to Red Tent. We stop to pick up a friend on the way and drive into town laughing and talking. The gathering this month is intentionally simple, a "cards and conversation" format of circle in which we eat a potluck dinner, share oracle card decks and layouts, and spend time casually in one another's company.

We circle for a brief meditative moment, dropping into our bodies and this space together. We pass the rattle, round, red, and owl-shaped, and do a brief check in about our lives. The mood remains light-hearted and jocular, without the tears so often prompted by the rattle. I tell them of my gratitude for my almost completely healed leg, my body's steady, devoted, tireless, incremental progress in getting better. We pair up in small groups, sharing cards, talking about ideas. I talk about writing and poetry with a poet-writer friend and find myself patting my heart with intensity talking about the drive and compulsion I feel to share what I write. She understands. I see the passion burning behind her own eyes as we take turns listening to one another and to that unquenchable fire from within that must be freed.

The evening is full of laughter and pleasure. It is a delight to feel so at ease together and to not be personally responsible for a significant event or a major plan, just the pleasure of one another's company in sacred space.

On the drive home, the last rays of sunset streak cherry fire in layers across the sky behind the trees. We straddle at least five toads hopping across the road, and at the mouth of the driveway in the last remnants of twilight we see Limpy and her twin fawns, alert and watchful, as we reach home.

Expansion...Contraction

The hawk cries at dawn and the rising sun makes a red ball in the corner of the bedroom window. *May you dwell in devotion, may you dance with dreams,* I wake thinking.

I walk alone in the stale and humid morning, feeling the itch for magic, the desire for *something more.* I am frustrated with myself for not *feeling it* today, for being ragged and frayed at my edges, uneasy in my mind, and pinched in my heart-space.

Finally, I sing my Persephone song and sink back into presence. I look at the last remaining purple flags of vervain, scouting for seeds to collect and pause at the sawtooth sunflowers to take photos, the multi-striped goddess shining peacefully in the sun. As I rise creakily from my squat, a flutter of movement catches my eye and I look to see eight large black and blue swallowtail butterflies waving over the thistles that are illuminated in the morning sun. The thistles still in shadow are untouched, but the glowing thistles are bobbing and swaying under the delicate feet and investigating proboscis of this crew of waving wings.

I offer my three breaths to Persephone, still wondering about point and purpose, intention, and next steps. There is a flutter and something tangles in my hair, a brown butterfly that lands on my stomach and waits there.

> *A breath from my belly, center of creation.*
> *A breath from my heart, center of compassion.*
> *A breath from my head, center of curiosity.*
> *May all be easy in my temple*
> *and may I dwell in devotion*
> *in this day.*

I think about dynamic tension and the balance between constriction and expansion. My mom comes to mind, the ways in which I've felt my choices constricted by her and what she wants for me or tries to steer me into doing and all the countless and invaluable ways she supports and encourages me, both are present in dynamic tension. *Perhaps you can't have the support without the constriction,* I muse, *can't spread your wings without also knowing how to contract them inward again.* I sit up and the butterfly lands on my hand as I write, its patterned orange and brown wings opening and closing, tongue extended and tasting my hand as it moves across the page. It is so light I can barely feel it, but there is a small coolness where its tongue touches, a tiny pulse where its body hovers above six thready legs. Yellow mulberry leaves twist through the air, catching the light.

While I have been taking downtime to rest in the Cauldron, to collect my resources, to build my reserves, to breathe and to be, I am beginning to feel tight and worried about our income. It is on me, on my shoulders, to build, promote, and engage with our community. In intentionally stepping back, in enforcing boundaries on my time and availability, our sales have taken an abrupt nosedive and I'm feeling responsible for that decline. It *is* on me to keep our business fed and healthy, supporting us as I nourish our community with my words, attention, and tenderness. I choose a few goddesses and sit on the deck listening to the *Burnout* book whilst taking photos for new shop listings. I keep struggling with myself over my twin desires, which are in opposition at the moment: to take a pause, and to keep our business thriving. I am tight and angry with myself for my incapacity to let it be *and* at my own incapacity to accept my current state of mind instead of agitating for and pushing for something different, something better.

Instead of practicing yoga or sitting down at my computer to write, as I wish to do, or going to the tiny temple for ritual and meditative communion with Persephone as intended when I woke up this morning, I walk on the elliptical, ironically continuing to listen to *Burnout,* as I create new item listings for the product pictures I took outside. I feel the warring sensation within my chest. I could be doing this differently. I could be holding myself differently, I could be treating myself differently, I could be working differently, and yet, I can't allow it for some reason, pushing myself in and down and *getting it done* so I no longer feel so insecure. I feel weirdly split inside, like I'm arguing with myself, defeating myself, crying out for myself, critiquing myself.

Finally, after hours of work and tumbling thoughts and making pumpkin muffins for my children, I gather myself, my books, my cards, my journals, and go to the tiny temple, where I envisioned settling this morning. I feel headachy and anxious, tired and defeated. I also feel like I know what is happening. In the book *Meditations for People Who (May) Worry too Much*, I read about the relationship between worry and adrenaline. Anne Wilson Schaef explains:

> *Worry is one of our favorite "triggers" for an adrenaline "high." In fact, worriers who become addicted to the high often begin to find "normal" day-to-day life rather boring...*

While my trigger is not exactly worry, it *is* overworking, is having "too much to do." As I've already discovered multiple times this year, when I am in an unfamiliar state of ease, of rest, I find myself casting around for the push, for the familiar tension, for the agitated unrest of perhaps not being able to "get it all done." I create it for myself like an addiction, a hit of overwork to remind me I'm here, to stoke my brain into overdrive, to recognize myself as worthy and valuable. It feels safer to be overwhelmed, overdone, overbooked, overcommitted. *Not* being maxed to the limit, pushed to the edge, feels dangerously calm, unpleasantly easy, worrisomely peaceful.

Now in the temple, disengaged from the never-ending needs of children, I lie flat on my back in the air conditioning and let the knots in my body unwind, let my brain smooth and ease. I open myself to Persephone, offering her my breath, my devotion, my not-knowing, my need. I felt like I would take a meditative journey with her today, sinking into next steps, but instead I find myself soothing and honoring my body, speaking kindly and tenderly to myself in appreciation and gratitude. Beneath me, under the floorboards of the temple, I hear the leaves rustling and an animal stirring. I believe there is a raccoon directly beneath me, only one sheet of plywood and a strip of carpet away from my body as she lets herself go from the rigid expectations and persistent patterns of the day.

> *Take a deep breath*
> *all the way down to your toes*
> *feeling gratitude*
> *for your beautiful,*
> *strong,*
> *amazing*
> *body.*

Let yourself sink
into the sensation
of wholeness,
in just who
and how you are
right now.
You are so brave.
You are so worthy.
You are so loved.

Enoughness

There is a light breeze stirring as I step out onto the road, easing some of the heavy wetness of the air and cooling the sweat collecting on my lip and streaking my cheeks. The sky is white-gray and overcast and both orange and blue butter-flies bob on the waving purple thistle heads.

I am thinking about enoughness and acceptance, knowing that despite the feel-good messages about always, always being enough, often we actually are not enough for someone or something. The true task, I find, is to be okay with that. To accept that we are sometimes not enough for someone else, that sometimes others are not enough for us and that if we can breathe into that understand-ing, perhaps it can ease and dissolve as well. There is no need to get trapped in proving our own enoughness, rather we might need to witness the ways we have "failed" to be enough and still move forward anyway, still exist anyway, still create anyway. There is a certain freedom in considering who I might have let down, disappointed, dissatisfied, and been not-enough for and then continue to walk by these thistles anyway, watching the butterflies and feeling the wind against my face.

Listen.
I am the sound of silence
in your own heart.
I speak of rest
quiet peace,

the answers that
come from within.
Shhhh....
Listen.

I turn over all the things I'd like to do with my Cauldron Time and none feel like the right things. *Why am I scared to really do it?* I wonder. *To do all the things I say I want to do, all the things I crave deep within, all the knowing I wish to uncover, all the mystery I feel brewing? Why am I scared to let myself* ***be?***

What do I actually want? Because when I make space for it, I feel disinterest and apathy or a sense of "waiting." It is as if the "not having time" response is an excuse or story, not a reality. I think about the dance between effort and ease, some kind of internal tension seems to be necessary to birth change, create, and to take steps.

I lie back and ask myself: *what do I actually want to do?*

I want to serve the Goddess.
I want to walk in devotion.
I want to witness and write.
I want to reach out and touch
the lives of others through
word and image.
I want to sink into being
wholly myself.

I want not just a few hours or scraps with which to "catch up," I want a radically restructured approach to how I move through my *whole life.*

As I sit in my tiny temple with an expanse of time today and find myself at a loss as to what to choose, I wonder if sometimes there is more inspiration to be found in the stolen moments than in a broad, uninterrupted, stretch of open space. I open some of my ritual kit materials and use a piece of obsidian for a cord cutting ritual, passing it around my head, arms, and shoulders as I trim away the sensation of obligation, the belief that it has to be hard to be worthwhile, the need to prove myself, the persistent sensation of responsibility for other people's thoughts, feelings, experiences, and needs.

I lie down for a Persephone meditation, but find my attention wandering. I try to make a list of future projects, ideas I have been tabling that I wish to breathe life and being into. Then, I go to talk to Mark and we have a moment of clarity: the studio is his big project this year. And this book is mine. We have our projects, our passion work, right now in front of us. The others can wait. Trying to accelerate myself, pushing to regain a sensation of overwhelm, struggling to add more projects so I once again experience my life, my work, as more than I can handle, is unnecessary. I have my big project already. I am steadily working on it every day. I am living and loving myself into it. *This is enough.*

The nearly full moon is high above the field, looking hazy and foggy behind slight drifts of cloud in the still daylight sky.

> *May I deepen into stillness.*
> *May I deepen into listening.*
> *May I deepen into trust.*
> *May I deepen into patience.*
> *May I deepen into presence.*
> *May I allow myself this space*
> *to deepen and renew.*

Creativity and Mothering

Alaina wakens us at 2:45 a.m. crying from bad dreams and loneliness. By the time we agree to let her sleep in our room, we've awoken too much to go back to sleep easily. There is lightning rippling outside the windows, producing a strobe-like pulse of light throughout the house. Distant thunder begins to rumble along with the nearly continuous lightning. As I lie awake staring at the pulsing night, the thunder advances and the storm rises and crashes in around us, whipping and thrashing. I hear a repeated message inside my head:

> *When silence settles, let it fall*
> *that is when the old ones call.*

I lie there for hours, replaying the message, trying to remember it, dozing and waking with the words rolling around my mind, shaping into a poem, a larger message. I finally sleep and with full awakening to the bright light of morning, the message slips away, though I heard it twining and insistent, and important, all night long. I get up and write anyway, but I know it isn't the poem I should have written.

Even though it is relatively early morning, the air is thick and hard to breathe outside, heavy with water. The deck is slicked with rain and dotted with fallen yellow leaves. The ground is satiated and can breathe once more. A sweet lilting birdsong fills the air and as I round the bend of the deck, circling through my morning prayers, I spot a bright, cheery red cardinal perched in the treetop singing merrily.

In the *Burnout* book, I am on the chapter on rest and I am pleased to learn that I am actually getting more rest and restful activities than most American women. This makes me worry briefly that people may find my musings in this book to be "whining," instead of appreciating what I have, which is a symptom of being immersed in what the authors term "Human Giver Syndrome," in which we act to punish those who fail to uphold the syndrome.

Mark takes the younger children out while I finish up the workday with two of our employees and then excuse myself to write in the seclusion of the bedroom while they finish the last of the day's work.

When I pass my daughter's and my shared doll collection on the way out of the door, I feel a pang of guilt and regret that we have only played with these dolls a few times during this year. She is growing rapidly and I'm losing my chances to play dolls with her. This has been a persistent specter for me too, the worry that I'm working too much and the children's lives are slipping past me in a haze of, "do this" and "don't do this," with not enough joy and laughter.

I think about how much my children want from me, particularly my daughter, and how hard I have struggled and how much tension I have felt throughout my parenting journey between parenting and "personing"—helping and serving and tending to my children, while also nourishing my own heart and soul and the things I need to thrive and feel fulfilled. *Why,* I wonder, *are parents supposed to "sacrifice" for their children, only so their children can grow up to have children of their own to sacrifice for? Wouldn't it make more sense for each generation to live rich, full, fulfilling lives, instead of carving themselves down and away and relying on their children to fulfill their own unlived dreams?* I've refused to carve myself away, even though I have felt intense pressure to do so. Despite messages and memes and feel-good advice books to the contrary, I do not think a sacrifice of full personhood is required to still be a present and connected parent.

I keep a quote from a *Meditations for Women Who Do Too Much* page-a-day calendar (Anne Wilson Schaef) on my desk in the tiny temple. It reads:

The greatest gift we can give our children is growing up with a mother who is becoming who she can be and taking care of herself in the process. This is, of course, also the greatest gift we can give ourselves.

My essay for *Feminism and Religion* was published this morning and I check my email to find a rash of positive responses to it that touch my heart and encourage me. I am heartened and encouraged to read the replies from other women, several of whom are authors I admire, and grateful they have taken the time to read my words and share their thoughts.

In the book *A Question of Balance: Artists and Writers on Motherhood,* Linda Vallejo, a Mexican-American artist known for her evocative paintings, is asked whether she feels guilty for going into the studio to paint. Her reply inspires me:

Why should I? I believe if you're given a gift, you must use it. If you have the gift of writing and poetry and beauty in any form — sculpture, painting, dance, music, literature, cooking, sewing, any of the traditional arts — you have a responsibility to the symbolic and physical whole to live it out.

In another interview in the book, poet Alicia Suskin Ostriker explains the psychic cost of combining writing and mothering:

I'm sure that many people will tell you this: Taking care of children is a tremendous drain on your time, your spirit, your feelings, your self-image, and there's no way around that. So that's the downside. The positive side is that having children keeps you real, keeps you open and on your toes and is a continuing learning experience. [It] gives your mind and your passions a constant workout — which, if you want to keep them alive, is not a bad thing to have happen.

And, finally, in an interview with Linda Hogan, she explains:

My writing precedes my thinking. I feel, in some ways, the writing is a teacher. I don't know where it comes from. I know that my writing is a lot more intelligent than I am... And, it's wiser than I am. So paying attention to the work is, in some ways, paying attention to the deepest part of my own self, my own spirit. I also feel that when I'm working well, the land itself speaks through me. I become the medium for a greater knowledge and a greater intelligence than just mine... You have to protect yourself as a writer, and you have to do your work. On some levels, the work is a part of spirituality, it's part of a deep soul growth, and to sacrifice it means you sacrifice your integrity and the honor of your own life and language.

Sometimes I feel like creativity is a fire I can't make space for, a demand I'm not big enough to fulfill, a battering wave, an endless tower, a full-blast faucet of uncontrollable inspiration. Creativity crumbles my human limits, believes in miracles, and refuses to be silenced, clawing its way madly from the bent lines and wild constraints of a human-sized life and demanding to be heard and held, asking, always asking to be so much MORE, ravenous for time, starving for silence, and ragged with need. It is sharp-edged and fierce, ferocious, and tenacious, worn at the edges and molten at the core.

I write to invite delight to rest in my bones, to let passion and wonder sing in my blood, and inspiration burn in my fingers, I write to let hope sear my soul and open my eyes. I write because sometimes I feel like I'm saving my own life with my words.

We walk too late, scurrying along in the deepening night and startling a brave bunny. The sun is setting round and red across the valley, in a manner similar to a sunset over the ocean, dropping straight beneath the straight line of horizon instead of sinking in stages behind the trees. We stand undecided for a moment at the driveway's end, deciding which direction to go, but I see a crow in the road and say, *Remember we are following the crows.* So, we first head right, to the northwest. The crow flies into a dead oak tree in the field and perches, scenically silhouetted against the red sky, watching the sunset with us.

I show Mark the surprising milkweed, the butterfly flower, and the curled furls of morning glory. Then, we hurry back the other direction, still wanting to get a full walk in even though it is growing dark. As we come up the slight hill by an abandoned field, the round, golden moon rising large on the horizon actually startles me. It is beautiful, alive, and glowing, hanging low and big, in the twilight. A deer is silhouetted in the road with the moon behind her and we stop and stare, entranced and *here.* While we don't intend to walk at this late hour, I love that we have watched both sunset and moonrise together on this day, each a timeless moment of beauty that will never happen in exactly this way again.

No one
will ask you to slow down and do less
except for your children
and the milkweed by the side of the road
that you almost didn't see.

Morning Glory

This is my bloodland, I awaken thinking. The air is cool and welcoming this morning, inviting me out to explore. I hesitate at the end of the driveway, poised at a point of indecision, when a crow lifts off from the road and soars into the treetops calling, perhaps, *this way.* The morning glories are tight-furled in the cool morning.

As I descend the hill, my nose prickles and I feel a distinct sensation of entering another world: sharp, alert, inhuman. I see the crow again, first one lifting from the road and then a second beyond it, swooping out of the tree and away into the forest, and then finally, the third, this one rising from a tree closer to me and taking flight, calling loudly. I follow them, careful and alert, my footsteps too loud on rocky ground, crunch, crunch, crunch. One crow continues to call just out of sight, loud and insistent, alarmed or informing, I'm not sure. I stop, looking into the woods for it, and a shape at the gravel's edge catches my eye and comes into focus, a long, thin vulture's wing feather, partially buried in the rocks and Virginia creeper.

I continue to walk as quietly as I can, the pileated woodpecker trills to my left and the crows continue their raucous caws to my right. I wonder if I am missing something, I am a sense-dull poor excuse for an animal, I think. The woods begin to crack and creak, alive with noise. It sounds like a hundred small things falling through countless leaves—acorns, hickory nuts, leaves, old raindrops, I cannot tell, but they continue to speak with a crunching sort of continuous sound, almost like a giant creature chewing in multiple directions.

Finally, I hear the cry of a red-shouldered hawk join the crows and decide to turn back. As I walk back up the hill, I feel I am emerging from a journey. I find a curved sickle of rusted metal on the road and then stoop to gather six fallen morning glory blooms, closed into small flames of pink. As I hold my gifts, I realize they are elemental, one from each Air, Earth, and Fire. *What if I find a snail shell right now from Water?* I think. *Wouldn't that be magical?* I imagine the story I will write, the poem I will weave from the real-life magic of this day, but though I walk slowly, peering intently at the ditch for a curved spiral of white or brown, I find nothing and I realize that in looking so hard, I'm missing everything.

> *If there is anything I've learned*
> *this year,*
> *it is that magic unfolds on its own,*
> *no forcing needed.*

Self-Sovereign

I don't have a lot of walking time today, so I move swiftly, feet squelching instead of crunching today, the gray chert on this part of the road forming a soft mud.

On the way back up the hill, singing my Persephone prayersong, I pause midway to greet the morning glories. I am thinking about how surprised I was to encounter Persephone in the first place, how I thought I would "switch" goddesses this year, how surprised that she's not finished with me...and I'm not finished with her.

I look back to the beginning of the year with amazement at how much more complex and lengthy a process of unraveling and rebuilding it has been than I anticipated, and how much further I suspect I have yet to grow. I offer my gratitude for her steadiness, for not letting me know everything yet, for not letting it be simple and tidy, and swift and surface, but requiring depth and digging and persistence. *Don't give up,* is one of her most consistent reminders to me when I continue to plead, *What's next? How do I know what the next step is?*

I think about how radically I underestimated her, dismissing her as a "victim" goddess or as too simplistically "maiden" for me, when she is really such a strong and tenacious goddess. Then, it strikes me, so sudden, so obvious: Persephone in *patriarchal* myth *is* a victim. She is objectified, possessed, controlled, but she actually becomes self-sovereign, ruling her domain, centered in her own power, potential, and purpose. While her story *begins* with force, it *ends* with *choice*, and a recognition of her own power.

I have been on an Underworld journey of choice versus force this year too, feeling victimized by my own schedule, commitments, family, out of control of my own life and then slowly, slowly rebuilding my own agency and coming to confront my own self-sovereignty, even as I have had to also confront how often I, myself, sabotage or undercut my own freedom of choice, my own sense of agency.

Persephone rises from victim to queen, holding her own in the deepest shadows and levels of being and becoming. She is misunderstood and minimized. I have also misunderstood and minimized her. She isn't who I would have picked to work with, but she is who I needed.

The Twelfth Task

You may choose
whether or not
to dance
with your life,
sunstreaked, awestriped,
ragged, and strong
on the changing edges
of a mysterious world.
This much is up to you.

I awake to a repeating refrain that chases all the morning prayers out of my head and leaves only this thought, lingering: *whether or not you choose to dance with your life — that much is up to you.* You can either dance with your life, or not. It all comes down to that.

I walk slowly, this time to the border of the dry creek where I discover a small cluster of skullcap flowers raising purple flags of wonder above the stones, the slightest tickle of raindrops kissing my shoulders. The air is thick and heavy, humid and hard to breathe already.

> *Be both tender and tenacious.*
> *Rise strong from where you have drifted.*
> *Heal where you can.*

I think about the river and about learning from Water. I feel like perhaps it will be the Fall Equinox that will usher me into learning from Water once more. I will go to the river and to the ocean and see what they have to teach. I've accepted that I will still be walking with Persephone for the remainder of the year, even if my elemental focus shifts to Water. I remember how I intended to visit the river at least once a week this year, but how that urge has faded or been replaced in priority with my road walks and temple time and the continued swirl of home and business, the never-ending advance of time and tasks.

I spot a lovely rippled red rock leaning scenically against a dead tree twined with Virginia creeper and I pause to take a picture, enjoying the way the goddess looks in this tiny landscape, as if she is on a mesa in Arizona instead of on a gravel roadside in Missouri. I think about the size of my life and if it is "too small." I like it this small: consciously cultivated, intentionally, mindfully structured into smallness, shrinking to the size of this stretch of road, my deck, our broad field. *This is my bloodland,* comes back to me, as I look at the brown and white goddess standing in the sunshine on a rusty red and rippling stone. *I can learn everything I need to know, right here.*

I begin to sing now, my body prayersong, feeling swept with gratitude for my moving, working legs on this uneven ground.

> *My body is my altar,*
> *my body is my temple,*
> *my living presence on this earth*
> *my prayer,*
> *my prayer,*
> *my prayer.*

I think about how *this,* this going out and exploring and returning with tales and experiences to share with others is my ministry, in this devotional practice, in this witnessing, in this attention to smallness, I reach out to touch the lives of countless others. In feeding my own devotion, in nourishing my own soul, I nourish so many more. *This is my work. It counts and it is real.* It doesn't mean I have it all figured out, or even that I have anything figured out, but that I am taking the time to pay attention, to listen, to witness, and share.

> *Some may say my world is too small,*
> *the size of a square deck,*
> *a field of waving grasses and wildflowers,*
> *a strip of brown and gray gravel road,*
> *a tiny temple shrouded in oak leaves,*
> *roses,*
> *and incense.*

I breathe deeply and wonder why it has been so hard to withdraw, to pull myself in, to lie on the floor, to be still and let myself bubble. I think about crouching in the morning glories, about sweat slicking my face in the blackberries, about a horsefly biting me in the center of my back as I look at yellow foxgloves. I think about the color of ripe poke and elderberries, the rising of a round golden moon, I think about the taste of wild blueberries. These things come from action, from doing, from being out and present *in the world,* not in retreat. It is in the messiness, the not-fun moments coupled with the awe, *that is where the story lives.*

What if I get out of my own way? Stop blaming myself or anyone else for block-ing me from what I desire and simply listen to desire and then do it, read it, write it, feel it, open it, create it, live it?

I can trust myself.

> *The twelfth task is:*
> *to get out of*
> *my own way.*

Space

The hawk cries at dawn, bringing me into wakefulness, but it has already silenced in the heat by the time I step outside at 7:30. Puffs of purple thistle are open by the deck and spirals of spider web glow in the new sun. Mark has laid spires of mullein on the gardening bench and before I walk, I decide to roll some of the leaves into tapers for later dipping into beeswax to burn. The sun is at my back, sweat already starting to roll down between my shoulder blades as I choose which leaves to roll. Many are riddled with insect holes, but they are soft and pliable beneath my fingers. *I see why they call it flannel plant, or blanket plant,* I think, as I roll. The leaves feel almost like fabric, they are strong and dense, while also puffy and soft. The small hairs on the leaves rub off onto my shirt as I hold them against my belly to roll them more tightly. I don't want to miss my chance to walk, but this is unexpectedly contemplative: quietly, deliberately, mindfully, rolling fuzzy leaves into tapers under a morning sky, in silence, no other tasks, worries, concerns or voices. The hawk's call rises again, once, twice, three times and I step out from under the green metal roof to try to see it, but it silences once more.

I roll thirty leaves in the quiet of the morning, lining them in neat rows on the back of the gardening bench, and then walk down the driveway heading towards the low, faded round of waning moon. I head right first, the sound of crows ringing distantly over my left shoulder, and check on the milkweed. Then, I cross back and go the other direction, where the road is flat instead of hilly, swinging my arms and singing. I am thinking about a devotional prayer book idea, turning over older writings and seeing how they could easily be adapted to fit many goddesses and personal practices. I feel inspired by the idea and excited to share it with others.

I round the corner and move briefly under the hot sun at the crossroads and then turn back, my two miles for the morning nearly complete. As I step along the last stretch of road before home, still singing, a small snake catches my eye, moving to the side just as my foot comes down. I am certain I have stepped on it, my heart pounding and shock rolling through me as I skip-hop over to the center of the road away from it. I turn to look behind me to see only a stick in the road, gray-black and innocent. I swear I saw it move. There is no more singing as I finish my walk, feeling startled out of my lulled trance.

I am listening to *Year of Yes* by Shonda Rhimes this week. In it she gives a commencement speech at Dartmouth where she encourages people to be *doers* instead of dreamers. There is a lot of truth to this. Mark and I are both fond of saying that the idea is less than 1% of the process, 99% is actually doing it. I am a doer, quintessentially, completely. My maternal grandparents *did* until they died.

I am learning that there is — there must also be — a place for drinking tea and dreaming and breathing quietly while the knots loosen. I am also learning that it is fully possible to feed myself, nourish myself, build myself while also reaching out to nourish others at the same time. It doesn't *have* to be either-or. I can do the things I need and love and value and wish for and dream of *and* I can reach out and share those with others: one does not have to deplete or extinguish the other. I think of all the opportunities I've said no to so I can preserve my slices of silence, of introspection, and peace. I think of all the discoveries I've made in those slices and how I have used them to touch the lives of other people around the world. I have no regrets. There is a *lot* of *do* in my world. *Do* isn't wrong or bad, but I am only beginning to recognize how much of my own doing has been unnecessary or even marginally self-destructive. I am no longer willing to do until it hurts, even if that means letting an opportunity and then another and another float past me into the many shadows of what will not be.

In Day Schildkret's book *Morning Altars,* he writes:

> *I share because no matter what is happening in my life, the worries of my day or the stress of my budget, I long to connect my heart to everyone else and to believe beauty is magic that can lead us out of our lonely story and back into the great togetherness that I know we are all craving. And I share because this is what we humans have always done, in every culture. We have created beauty as a way back to remembering ourselves, as a way of getting through the hard times, as a way of taking care of each other and of speaking the language of soul, myth, Earth, and magic.*

What I need, what I was missing when I began this journey five months ago, is *space,* margin for simply living, for feeling the rain, for photographing the flower, for watching the crow soar overhead, and for hearing the messages in these experiences so I can share them with others.

As I move my computer from the temple to the workroom so I can start preparing orders for tomorrow, I listen to an audio from the writer's Oasis offered by Jennifer Louden. She quotes Thomas Merton from his book *Conjectures of a Guilty Bystander.* It is a quote I recognize from years ago, I used to keep it taped to my laptop:

There is a pervasive form of contemporary violence to which the idealist most easily succumbs: activism and overwork. The rush and pressure of modern life are a form, perhaps the most common form, of its innate violence. To allow oneself to be carried away by a multitude of conflicting concerns, to surrender to too many demands, to commit oneself to too many projects, to want to help everyone in everything, is to succumb to violence. The frenzy of our activism neutralizes our work for peace. It destroys our own inner capacity for peace. It destroys the fruitfulness of our own work, because it kills the root of inner wisdom which makes work fruitful.

We walk at dusk and turn back early in the heat and the rapidly growing darkness. Above the field, a bird flaps across our path sudden and erratic, darting and zipping in a manner similar to a bat. It has distinct stripes of white under its wings that catch the last of the fading light. It is a nighthawk, the first we've ever seen and we are entranced and blessed to watch it, busily attending to its work.

> *May you find a place for wandering.*
> *May you find a place for witnessing.*
> *May you find a place where you are whole and held.*

Migration

May you know when to step forth gleaming, eyes alight and ribbons streaming.

Rain falls most of the night and by morning, a fresh wave of storm lashes across the sky. Thunder rolls and the ground is drenched, the sky a monotonous sweep of bright gray. I cannot go for my morning walk, so I sit in the temple shrouded in both a cocoon of silent stillness and the persistent sound of rain on the roof. I miss walking and discovering, but instead I make a fifteen-minute audio for my *Living the Questions* program about witnessing without fixing and what I mean when I use that phrase.

Sometimes there is no poem in the air or on the rain. Sometimes we feel parched and wandering. Sometimes we feel oversaturated, awash with our own feelings and needs, or flooded with the needs of others so that our own needs are drowned out. Sometimes we feel dry and cut off. This is all part of the landscape of living.

We are getting ready to leave for a short mini vacation to Table Rock Lake, three hours away. There is a mound of work to do to close up the shop for this break and to pack the things six people need in order to travel, including food.

I lie on the floor for my breaths:

Persephone, I am open to your guidance. I am open to what is.

Am I?

I am open to your process. I am open to your purpose. I am open to your path.

After dinner we walk under a deep gray sky lit with small patches of glowing yellow and magenta. As we come up the slope where the brave bunny usually sits, it runs from us, and we see a few birds swoop swallow-like over our heads. They are larger than swallows though and we become aware that there are many of them, flying in a wave, intent with purpose. A ball of glowing dusky pink sits on the horizon like a sunset, but in the East, mysteriously. The clouds are thick and smoky, dipped and swirled and curled in a dramatic vista as the birds stream past. We stop in the middle of the road, transfixed, looking up where we see the telltale white stripes across the underside of each wing. It is a nighthawk migration and we are here to see it, the exact right moment, the exact right road, the exact broad field, the exact heavy sky. There are at least fifty birds, each passing in the swath of sky above our heads, silently, purposefully, magically. As quickly as it began, it is over, the last bird cresting the treetops and away and we are left in the road, grounded in awe at what we have been privileged enough to see.

May you know when it is time
to cocoon with purpose.
May you know your own heart
as worthy and true.
May you trust your own voice to
speak your story into being.
May you rely on your steady steps
to guide your way.
May you weave a basket of wonder
to hold the precious blossoms of your dreams.
And may you trust your own essential goodness
today and all days.

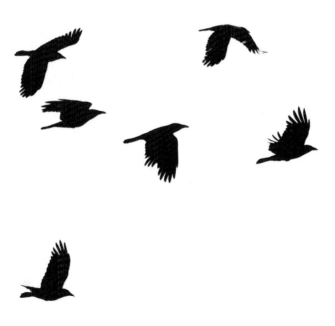

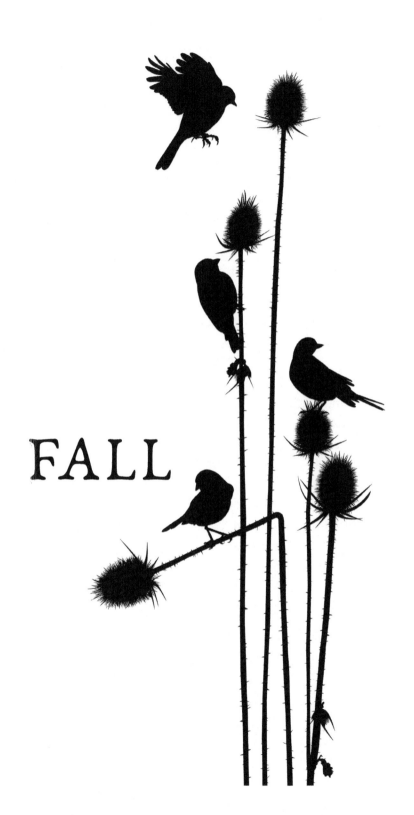

FALL

SEPTEMBER

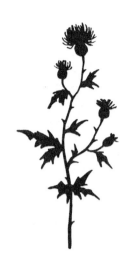

New Moon in Fog

It is misty and cool outside, a white fog hanging over the field and the barest whisper of drizzle falling. I reach the end of the driveway and look both ways to choose where to go. I am surprised to see three crows rise up silently to the left and soar away across the trees. For the first time, I turn away from the crows and instead follow the mist, down the hill and into the bottomlands, into an Underworld of my own mind.

My mom drives by, on her way to clean at the river cabin. She stops and we talk briefly on the road, me in the ditch, her in her blue SUV. My dad follows shortly behind on his blue tractor, heading to the river to mow before our family and friends potluck dinner plan tomorrow afternoon.

I feel pulled out of my private exploration, the solace of solitude. Having to turn on, to smile, to laugh, to make conversation, to be interested. I feel the mask of pleasantness settle onto my face, so familiar that it is almost unnoticeable. But then I think that I don't want to be pleasant. I don't want to be nice, to talk. I feel as if I have to be "on" so often, there is no rest from pleasantness, from engagement, from smiling. *Isn't this the price of connection though?* I wonder. *Doesn't only doing what you want and feel or is easy drive away relationship, weaken the fibers of connection, undermine the threads of love?*

I squeeze through the gate and walk down the driveway toward my parents' lodge building, this log cabin perched on the hill overlooking the valley. Bright blue chicory is blooming along the sides of the road. I part some of the grasses surrounding it and kneel down for photos. Through the fog of my headache, a message from chicory begins to twine in my dulled and pain-streaked brain. I think about its use as a coffee substitute and wonder: *What if you refuse to accept yourself as a substitute, but honor the fullness of who you really are?*

> *Bloom while you can.*
> *Trust your roots.*
> *Turn your face to the sun.*
> *Do not settle for being a substitute,*
> *honor the fullness of who you are.*

I leave the chicory and stop by the purple asters, dipping low by the brown gravel, orange-yellow eyes bright in their centers even on a gloomy day. Beyond the flowers I see the red glint of rosehips and I almost reach out to pluck some when I recognize the green berry clusters and coloring leaves of the abundant poison ivy in front of them. When I stand and continue up the hill the white-frosted gleam on the skin of a purple-red, unripe persimmon catches my eye. I pick it up and carry it home.

A swoop of wings shadows my path and I look up to see a vulture rise from the trees right next to me and circle away above my head. It is so close I hear the soft, whispering rustle of its wing feathers. It circles three times, obviously trying to come back to its position, but I am too slow at moving on my way and it drifts away. I am surprised to see another one still sitting, hulking black against the sky. Our eyes meet and it too lifts off and glides away from me, wings whispering as they rise and fall. I labor up the hill and as I reach the top, I see the vultures have moved there instead, sitting dark and forbidding in a dead tree near the neighbor's pond. *You can always choose which way to go,* they remind me.

On the back deck, I open my journal, feeling the dim whisperings of a poem struggling to rise up from my pain-fogged brain. There are words wanting to twine and twirl, to be woven into being. There is wisdom here. There are vultures on the wing and chicory in bloom. I know there is something to be said. The sky is a bright, deep white as I sit motionless, pen in hand, waiting for the words slowly bubbling to the surface from their Underworld of pain.

It has been twelve weeks since I fell and in those twelve weeks, I have only had a headache bad enough to warrant taking an ibuprofen twice. This is a dramatic change for someone who has experienced chronic headaches since puberty.

Today, I woke with a familiar film of pain behind my eyes. It feels as if there is an actual sheet of something foggy layered between my brain and the front of my skull. I feel fuzzy and dulled, almost feverish, as if I am just moving through my day while separated from it by this layer of pain. I have the sensation that my soul has wandered away from my body and I am left behind, dull and grasping. I finally cave and take the ibuprofen after lunch. I didn't want to give in, didn't want to break my record, didn't want to admit I can't cope with it, and yet, it lingers.

I do yoga. I try to journal. I feel flaccid and stale. I take another one at 4:30, waiting for my spirit to come back to me. I recognize my feelings of pointlessness, despair, worthlessness, disinterest as signs of this fog of pain. I know from experience and have already even written in this book about this sensation. It isn't actually real. It is an artifact of pain. When the headache finally lifts, my spirit, my inspiration, my sense of purpose will reconnect to me, I just have to wait.

I try to soften into it, sink into it, witness without fixing. It is against my core nature to be "dull," however. I find this lifelessness nearly unbearable. I let the dullness wash over me, settle in. I go to the tiny temple and arrange myself on the floor and lie down, hands open at my sides, eyes closed. I offer my breaths to Persephone, slowly and intentionally, and then I sing.

Since I feel alone and safe, I sing full-throated and loud, I let my voice rise high and sink low in waves, I feel surrounded by my song. As it fades away, I let myself drift, my edges dissolving, my limbs becoming heavy, my sense of my own body's borders fading away. I invite Persephone to show me next steps and she says:

You already know. Wait. Watch. Write.

I rouse myself from my meditative stillness, my deconstructed sensation of bodily presence and step outside the temple, barefoot on the earth. Two crows caw loudly from the trees beside me and I smile.

My headache finally fades at dinner time, my spirit and smile returning, my ability to make plans, have ideas, and feel creative slowly flowing back into me. I can feel all these parts rejoining, reconnecting, reigniting, and I am grateful.

We walk at dusk under dark and cloudy skies. A quiet brown deer is on the shoulder of the road in the rosehips and poison ivy. After studying us for a few minutes, it runs too. We walk back home with Mark's flashlight trained at the road looking for snakes. Sunset is coming earlier and earlier and our walking plans will need to adapt.

I chose not to follow crows today,
but turned away
to follow the mist instead,
descending down a rocky hill
and into an Underworld of my own making,
I was reminded that we can always
choose which way to go,
and that even thin and tattered magic
is worth
savoring.

Sing Louder

Life is an unfoldment, and the further we travel the more truth we comprehend.
To understand the things that are at our door is the best preparation for
understanding those that lie beyond.

—Hypatia

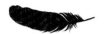

I rise early, moving through my prayers quickly and with half a brain, the other half lost to distraction. There is a thin white film of mist across the hills. The sound of crows fills the valley. I take only a few steps down the road when a great hawk skims impossibly low over the grasses, white underbelly almost touching the green spears. It alights gracefully in the tree where I saw it before. I pause, breathless, jolted from my whirling thoughts and to-do lists, watching it. As soon as it sees that I am still moving forward, it lifts its broad wings again and swoops out of sight into the trees.

I come inside singing softly to myself, going to the workroom to write for a few minutes before leaving. Tanner hears me and says, *Oh, mama! What is that beautiful song? Sing louder!* I think this is the first time in my life I've been asked to sing louder, as music and vocal talent has never been one of my gifts.

I think of all the women at Red Tent who I have led through countless songs, many reluctant at first, but then voices rising together. I am self-conscious of my own tendency to sing off key or to vary the melody unpredictably as it suits me, but somehow, we have an entire SoundCloud album of us singing, together, because I've been willing to look past shame and keep singing.

I remember listening to an interview with David Hillman on Karen Tate's *Voices of the Sacred Feminine* podcast. He stated that when political and religious tides were turning in the ancient world, those who wanted to dominate and control others didn't go for the leaders of countries, for political heads of states, or for those in powerful jobs, they went for the priestesses. They went for the women who held the cultural stories and ritual language of the people. They went for the healers and nurturers and those who took care of others. They destroyed temples and sacred images and books. They almost succeeded in total eradication of the role of priestess from the world and worked really hard to take midwives and wise women out completely as well. While I may not have often been literally asked to "sing louder" in my life, I have woven countless ceremonies, sacred experiences, and community into being using my words, my breath, my voice, and my hands. This is, in its own way, my way of singing louder.

It is that holy poetry and singing we are after. We want powerful words and songs that can be heard underwater and over land. It is the wild singing we are after, our chance to use the wild language we are learning by heart under the sea. When a woman speaks her truth, fires up her intention and feeling, staying tight with the instinctive nature, she is singing, she is living in the wild breath-stream of the soul. To live this way is a cycle in itself, one meant to go on, go on, go on.

—Clarissa Pinkola Estés

Trance-ported

I wake early, alert and interested, expecting a discovery. The sunrise is flaring bright and orange and there is a linger of promise in the air. I slip quietly outside into a cool morning. For a moment I think I can see a puff of my own breath in the air. There is a huge spider web strung gracefully between the porch rail and mulberry tree.

I stand in the light of sunrise, opening my hands to the new day. The air is fresh and cool and sweeps over me.

The sound of crows rises wild and near, filling the woods on three sides of me. I move quietly over to where one is in the trees behind the raspberries. It participates in a sort of call and response back and forth with a crow deeper in the trees, unseen, in the deep gully behind the house.

> *I am in love*
> *with the wild grasses*
> *of morning*
> *and the way sunlight*
> *rests on seed and stem.*

I move further down the road, called by the glowing plumes waving gently under the blue sky, pops of yellow and purple blooming behind them, my eyes on the golden fronds. I am enthralled, enchanted, transported...trance-ported.

I don't even realize how immersed I am in the sun on the seeds until I emerge from the trance, shaking my head a little, feeling dizzy and completely alive. This immersion in complete focus, sinking totally into the present is like traveling into another realm, another plane of experiencing. It is the first time I've become so wholly and totally present, completely aware, completely soft and *here,* since my morning glory morning walk last month. I pause in the road and almost shake myself, bringing myself back into functioning, normal human awareness and out of expansive trance-portation. I kneel to take pictures in the graceful bending stalks of wild rye, stretching over the brown-eyed Susans, and then turn back, feeling as if I'm emerging from an Otherworld of being as I step along the rocks. I see purple stands of poke stem gleaming in the woods by the rocks where I used to sit with such devotion. Bugs creak in the air. I face the sun and let the wind sweep my shoulders.

I am holding a fierce truth.
This benediction of fierceness forms and moves through me.
I pick a perfect green acorn up off the rocks and carry it home.

> *May I follow my fierce inspiration.*
> *May I trust my fierce longings.*
> *May I explore my fierce curiosity.*
> *May I embrace my fierce devotion.*
> *May I love with fierce passion.*
> *May I rest with fierce courage.*
> *May I give with fierce discernment.*

Walking into my Shadow

I wake early, the bright glow of the sun lighting the bedroom and a cool breeze from the window beckoning. A red-shouldered hawk is calling very near and insistent and I ease the door open and creep quietly outside. The heat has finally broken and the air is brisk and cool. I stand silently behind the mulberry tree, listening to the hawk. It is right in front me, I can tell by the sound, but as I step out of my hiding place to try to see it, all I see is the barest shadow of wings lifting off and the cries of the hawk as it descends away from me, deeper and deeper into the trees and out across the valley.

I stand at the end of the driveway for a few moments looking both ways, deciding which way to go. I decide I don't want to navigate the hill today. The air is heating up. I feel sour and crabby, almost angry, about preparing for the Red Tent retreat, feeling used up, extinguished and fed upon as I have too often this year. This is not the spirit in which I wish to priestess and I wonder, again, if I have reached the end of this stage of my work in the world.

As I reach the crossroads, the wild grasses are lit with an ethereal, magical glow and I feel my spirits brightening with them. I step around them holding goddesses in my palms, between the stalks, the seeds, the light, feeling focused and alive. I circle the patch of grass and flowers and then head for home, my steps quick, my shadow black in front of me. *I am walking into my shadow,* I think.

I wonder about Medusa suddenly, if she is ready to come forward now, at this time. I think about my quick flares of anger, my need to reclaim my power and agency, and I wonder if I need her too. I realize abruptly that I haven't heard much from Persephone this month, that I've forgotten several days in a row to sing my prayersong on my walks. I wonder if this too, is an indicator of change. I think back to the Spring Equinox and the dramatic, palpable presence of Persephone in the winds by the lake. I haven't had a deeply magical experience like that in quite a while, I reflect.

As I turn into the driveway I stop in disbelief. A gigantic snake is stretched across the length of the road, black, green, and gold in the rays of sun. I am stunned. I squat down to look at it. Its head lifts and curves around slightly and then it slinks gracefully away and into the grasses of the field.

As I stand back up, feeling shaky and glittering with the direct intensity of this communication, I realize that it is nearly the Fall Equinox. This is the time of Persephone's descent, her retreat, the time in which she withdraws from the world. I met her in the spring time and she has guided my steps for six months now, perhaps the second half of the year is raising its head, alert for something new. It is not lost on me that the experiences of this day feel as if they were birthed from a literal crossroads, light and shadow meeting in one.

Red Tent

I get to the lodge early to clean before the women arrive. I've asked for volunteers to help early with the set up, but no one comes. Feeling tight and tired, I settle into the rhythm of wiping down the tables, cleaning the sinks, sweeping up the abundance of dead wasps, moths, and ladybugs that have collected along the walls and windowsills. As I sweep, I think about the snake in the road and Medusa. I think about my prayer to her, *Medusa, please rise through me,* and how it doesn't rhyme tidily like my Persephone song, so I start to mentally dance with the words. I cast off the idea of trying to get anything to rhyme with "uh" and instead think of how I can expand my greeting to include a rhyming word. As with the Persephone song that bubbled up and out of me during a beach walk, I feel the correct choice of words being handed to me. "Rage" is rejected in favor of "fury" and the verse becomes:

Medusa of fury and stone,
please rise through me,
in heart and bone.

I start to sing aloud as I swipe down cobwebs, reaching into every corner.

There is an enormous spider web strung across the front door, nearly filling the entire opening with the spider centered in the middle. I gently disconnect the anchoring threads and move the spider into the flowers. A friend arrives and takes over the task of chipping the wasp nests out of the doorway. Another friend hangs up my goddess banners and vacuums, freeing me to lay out the altar space and set up our central goddess grid for our ritual. I work carefully on the grid, since I have time to devote to building it with thoughtfulness and intention. I place green glass leaves and acorns and hematite keys. Tiny goddesses in fall colors fill in the center and I border the design with carnelian and citrine. The room fills with women, they've all come.

We begin the retreat with a compliment circle during the rattle pass. Inspired by Shonda Rhimes in *Year of Yes,* I ask each woman to speak of what is going right for her, what she is proud of, what she is doing so well and wisely. Though each month I attempt to consciously steer us away from doing so, there remains a tendency in a women's circle with closely built connections that span years, to connect and bond over our shared difficulties, our struggles, our personal setbacks, strains, stresses, and failures. Though I tell the members of the circle and train other facilitators to recognize that Red Tents are not therapy groups and are not intended for extensive therapeutic "processing," there can be a tendency to slip into those patterns. This time, I encourage the women to reach into bravery and courage, and dare I say, satisfaction with themselves, their gifts, their skills, work, and offerings in this world. Today, we begin our circle with the tender spaces that are blooming. It is beautiful and we are left with a sense of power and smiles. After each woman has a chance to speak, some for the first time in this circle setting, I open the floor to complimenting one another. The kind words and affirming statements come easily, gifted to each other with authentic affection and tender regard. I am grateful I chose to set this tone for our time together and my heart is buoyant and full as we sing our Sanctuary song together and then break for the next part of our retreat.

We split into two groups, half sitting on the deck outside to make brooms, the other half inside in the kitchen making wool felted journal pens at the table. The air is still pleasant outside, the sun bright, but a breeze moves through us and our broom corn on the shady porch. It is delightfully witchy to bind brooms on a nearly fall day with my friends and though I blister my finger in the process, I am enchanted by this world I've created around me, these connections forged with time and care.

We finish our handiwork and snack before moving to the back yard for a mini belly dance lesson from an experienced member of the circle. We adorn ourselves with jewelry and hip scarves and stand barefoot in a circle on the clean green grass. A small gray fence lizard moves out of our way across the porch as we begin. Our friend is clear about the ancient art and powerfully religious, goddess-honoring origins of belly dance, cautioning us away from viewing it as a titillating sparkly burlesque-type of experience, and sinking us into our bellies, our centers of power, of movement, of agency, of life. I am standing next to her, facing the others and as she speaks to us, I suddenly turn around to face the woods, where I am just in time to see a hawk swoop silently from the trees and pass along the outskirts of our circle, low, at eye-level, looking right at us as it glides past and into the woods beyond. We are speechless with amazed delight. I am so grateful I turned in time to bear witness to this gift of guardianship, of benediction. Immediately following the hawk, a bright orange butterfly dances around our circle. We relish these two gifts we receive this afternoon, barefoot on the grass, hips jingling with our dormant power.

We share stories in smaller circles then and then reconfigure in the kitchen for our shared meal. There is nothing like eating good food with a group of friends who have shared new experiences and power with one another. I feel incandescent with the connection we have built upon this day.

As the day shifts toward evening and the sun starts to lower across the horizon, we build a nature mandala together in the front yard, overlooking the valley. We lay out our brooms in the four directions, around a centerpiece of clam shells and druzy quartz surrounded by bright yellow wild sunflowers. We scatter bay leaves and jasmine flowers, sprigs of yarrow and branches of wild flowers and grains in a border around the edges of our wheel. It is huge and beautiful. We are grinning with wild delight at what we have built together. We gather for a group photo and then circle around for our whispered affirmations. We whisper to each other in nested circles and I feel the tears rise in my eyes as I hear the words of my friends forming a cone of sound around me. The affirmation I write for others is: *You are so inspiring.* The affirmation I receive to read to the women in the inner circle is: *You keep the stars. Smile. You are strong.* I whisper it to them, my hands resting lightly on the shoulders of each woman in turn. We then form a tunnel with our arms and say *I see you* as each woman passes under the arms of everyone else and takes her place around the mandala. This is unintentionally creepy when offered in our whispery voices and we end up dissolving into gales of laughter as we become progressively more creepy with each whispered pass. Instead of undermining the power of the ritual, it heightens and deepens it, bringing us into greater affection for one another, greater joy, and lighter hearts.

We call out what we are letting go of with each declaration lifting our arms in a great whoosh to let it fly away. Behind us the sound of frogs begins to rise out of the pond as the sun sinks lower in the sky and as we are serenaded by this great croaking, we sing.

The ritual ends with one of my own prayers of blessing. I am brave enough now to use these in circle without explanation or justification, and I offer the words with heart and love. This has been a powerful, magical day: my heart is full, my spirit strengthened, my resolve renewed. This work matters. And I am good at it. No longer do I feel slightly bitter and resentful, instead I feel woven into a tapestry of shared magic, of sisterhood, of song, of laughter, and the genuine delight of being alive together, hand in hand, on green grass beneath the sun-streaked sky.

After cleaning up and packing the car, I drive home in the now darkness, feeling buoyed up, reconnected, re-inspired, and re-enthused. I am bubbling with energy and excitement and happiness, exactly how I want to, and really should, feel after a ritual experience.

Mark and I walk on the deck as the orange moon begins to rise through the trees and I tell him about the gift of the hawk. He, in turn, tells me that after I drove away this morning, he found a complete shed snakeskin in the driveway behind my car. I am stunned into silence. *How could this be?* While I do wish I would have found it myself, the symbolic connection is still powerful enough to take my breath away.

Circles

I said I would know when it was time to finish. And I think I do. I began this book with a circle of women witnessing my truth, my ragged, worn, tired self. It ends now too, with a circle of women, full of laughter and song and joy of co-creation as a hawk glides before our eyes and we are witnessed once more into being.

I set forth to write myself back into wholeness in these pages, to rebuild my soul, to restore my joy. I have steadily, consistently, unfailingly continued to walk with the goddess and my soul across the days of six full months on the land on which I find myself.

I know, suddenly and with purpose, that I will end this volume with a ritual in the Underworld canyon of the land across the road on the Fall Equinox. And, with that ritual, a final poem will come. Not a permanent final poem, but the poem that will signify the conclusion of this book, this part of my journey.

A pale white moon nearly full hangs over the driveway as I begin to walk, the caws of crows echoing across the trees from the deep woods and valleys.

There is a tiny gray lizard on the road and beyond it I spot a small ring-necked snake. I bend down to meet its eyes, uncertain if it is alive or not, so still it is across the gravel.

Your whole life is a story, I think. *May it be a conscious, alert, alive, and centered one. May you notice sunlight on wild grasses and the shadow of silent wings across your path.*

I walk home into my tall, lean shadow until the road curves and I am now walking alongside my shadow as she stretches from the rocks of the road into the grasses of the field. As I turn into the driveway, I feel a sense of distance and calm, a sensation of settling within. Persephone is withdrawing for the year, not gone, but pulling away and handing me over to the next chapter. I stand by the railing on the deck, feeling a hollowed out sensation in my pelvis, an open channel, a sense of completion. A gray and white kingbird with a yellowish belly swoops into the air by my head and then a second one hovers ever so briefly in the tree in front of me, looking at me with black eyes before darting away.

May you make a space for tender wondering, I think, as I watch them fly away.

I circle the deck a few times to finish my two miles and think:

I am on fire with creation all the time. It is intense, pervasive, and persistent.

I have been listening and I do know that I'm done. It is finished as quickly, suddenly, and surprisingly as it began. And the poem comes...

> *May you make a space for wondering,*
> *carving it out of hollows*
> *between root and stone.*
> *May you make a space for wandering,*
> *ranging over lands*

striped with sunlight and shadow.
May you make a space for witnessing,
learning from wild grasses
and silent wings.
May you make a space for magic,
as she threads enchantment
through your bones and veins.
And, may you come to trust forever
the whispered spells
that weave and waver
right beneath
the tender knowing in your skin.

The Final Task

I walk on the driveway, feeling a sensation of closure, a sensation of openness. I feel like my noticing itself has changed texture. There is a tiny ring-necked snake in the road that I escort to safety with a little stick. The sumac leaves are turning red, dotted among the still green foliage and dust-covered leaves of the other plants and trees. I pause for pictures in the wild rye, the remaining sunflowers, the sunlight, and the sumac.

The final task is:
keep listening.

As I approach the driveway, I see a lone deer in the field across from me, eyeing me warily, large ears swiveled to face me, tail flicking. I slow my steps and turn quietly into the driveway where I see hoof prints in the dust.

Leave Taking

I dream of walking and finding two crow feathers in my path. I pluck them up with wonder and surprise that this magic is still waiting for me to discover it, to notice it, to let it bless me.

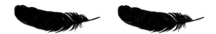

It feels like an important dream and it wakes me repeatedly throughout the rest of the night, my dream-self telling other dream people about these crows and how I need to remember them.

My sensation of having completed my work with this book is strong within me. It isn't that I'm no longer listening or no longer paying attention, but that my need to write down my experiences has ebbed and faded away.

Our oldest son, Lann, turns sixteen today. Born at sunrise on an equinox morning, this baby re-forged me into someone new, stronger, more tender, wiser, fiercer, and wilder than I had been before. I can hardly believe he is sixteen, the same age I was when I started to date his father.

Mark and I talk briefly in bed before getting up, remembering how this small baby fit along the length of Mark's thigh, sleeping with his dark hair swooping from its double crown, full lips relaxed, small hands soft and open. I remember the tender vulnerability of new motherhood, feeling split open and wounded, raw and exposed, deconstructed and rebuilt. Tears rise in my eyes as I remember him as our small one and thinking of all we've done to get him to here.

My blood begins today and it is time for my closing ritual with Persephone. It is time in my body, it is time in my page count, it is time in her rhythms, it is time in my spirit. After presents and a birthday breakfast, I practice yoga feeling restless and anticipatory. I pack up my little bag of ritual supplies, but I delay my departure by reading things on social media about climate change and the march for climate action. *There is so much to care about all the time,* I think.

I need to do this.
I am scared to do this.
Maybe I should wait.

I feel a sense of apprehension and I stall, reluctant to leave the house and to take this step.

I dab some of my blood onto a line drawing of a goddess outline. Around the edges I write the words to my Persephone prayersong in pink ink. The blood makes a heart shape of its own accord. I pack a vial of pomegranate juice, a bar of dark chocolate, a packet of dried flower petals. I pick two roses, one by the house and one by the new studio.

I think about the equinox, about balance, and centering.

May you be as balanced as butterfly, I think,

Expanding and contracting as needed to keep yourself aloft.

May you be as poised as a stone, letting the river part around you as it flows.

May you be as stable as a tree, flexing in the wind, while roots anchor deep below,

capable of charting the course of rivers and civilizations.

May you find the center from which you grow,

action and stillness,

listening and speaking,

waiting between worlds, between breaths, between days, between thoughts,

while sunlight and shadow meet.

Finally, I leave.

My sense of apprehension and unease persists as I step off the road and move through the trees, heading to the gulch where water over eons has cut a steep divide between the hills. It is full of craggy stones, slabs and boulders, tumbled together by the slow, inexorable forces of time and rain. The woods are silent. I see no birds and hear no crows. It is the heat of the day and I feel uncertain that this is the *right* time to be going and yet I also know,

I need to do this.

I step over crunchy moss, my eyes fixed on my feet, alert for snakes. This is the first time I've walked deep in the woods since I fell and hurt my ankle and I am amazed and grateful to be here again today, moving nimbly over this difficult and uneven ground. I remember myself three months ago, looking back at the woman who hops gracefully and surely from stone to stone and marveling that it was even possible to do so, possible to read the terrain so skillfully, possible to move with such assurance, with such certainty and confidence that my feet will bear me up and carry me forward. Now, here I am again, capacities restored, ankle a bit achy as it maneuvers, but skillful and capable once more.

I do not feel the sense of softening and settling that I often feel in the woods, however, the sense of "coming into myself," of being wholly present, alert and aware. Instead, I feel cautious, guarded, alert for danger rather than alert to wonder.

I navigate down the gulch, moving carefully across the slabs and dips of stones and old leaf cover, until I reach the ravine, the valley between two steep hills. Here, quiet descends. I have reached the Underworld I was seeking. The boulders are massive and covered with moss. The stones are silent. I finally feel my shoulders soften and my sensation of risk relax and ebb away. Now that I am not on steep terrain, I feel more secure. I also feel like I'm waiting for something, a sense of urgency within me, both to get back home for birthday dinner plans, but also, *to see this through.*

I turn east now and head up the ravine, seeking the location I found in my dream where Persephone, Queen of the Underworld, descended to me in a blaze of red and black. I realize with all my packing of supplies that I've forgotten to bring something to sacrifice, even though my dream indicated a sacrifice would be needed. *My book,* I realize. It is the laying down of my finished book that I have come to offer up, to see through. I look down and find a rock with a perfect hole through it at my feet. I pick it up and carry it with me.

I feel eager now, anticipatory, as I move more quickly along the rocks, seeking the place from my dream where the ritual will unfold. I follow my instincts, the guidance from within, even as time passes and I know I have somewhere else to be: I will keep walking until I know I am in the right spot.

Finally, I approach the tall white sycamore at the bend where two ravines meet. As I step onto the stones by the tree, the wind picks up and sweeps around me, blowing my hair back and curling around my arms. I feel like a character in a movie as it whirls around my body, like magic is all around me, the forces of the elements gathering into my hands. I feel the urge to go a little further and each time I stop, the wind whirls again, caressing and welcoming me. I clamber up the rocks and roots to where a shallow pool is formed in solid stone, water dripping steadily down the terraced stones, even though it hasn't rained in more than a month. Drifts of delicate blue wild skullcap drape from the stones, yearning toward the water.

This is it.

I settle myself on the leaves, by a slab of stone, facing the small pool, looking up at the pine trees and looking at a river of stony ground to both my left and right. I place my rock with a hole in it on the stone by my shoulder. This is Persephone's ground. I have descended. I have arrived. I lay out my ritual supplies and begin to speak. As I do, a bullfrog begins to croak from the pool. And I sense Persephone visually, though without literally seeing her. She is standing on the hill to my left, looking over her shoulder at me, golden hair cascading down her back, a robe across her shoulders. She steps away from me, shining light flowing from her fingers and trailing across the hills as she leaves. Our work together in this form, is finished. Her time here, in this way with me at this time of year, is complete.

> *We are balanced*
> *at the centerpoint*
> *of change,*
> *the stillpoint*
> *between breaths,*
> *the crossroads*
> *of being,*
> *watching as Persephone*
> *draws away,*
> *trailing golden light*
> *across the hills*
> *and the earth exhales*
> *before the deepening*
> *begins.*

The water continues to trickle down the stones. I pluck three hairs from my head and lay them across the leaves and I speak aloud, the words of my ritual and my gratitude.

Persephone, I have come today, journeying into your Underworld, into my
dream, in gratitude and appreciation for what we have wrought together over the
last six months. I am still yours and I will be yours as long as you will have me.
I am thanking you for the work that has come through me this year,
for the song, for the devotional prayerbook, for the magic of place,
for re-enchanting my world, rewilding my life,
for opening me up to a sense of mystery and majesty and magic
that is so much bigger and broader and more meaningful
than anything I ever imagined or dreamed of
and that can be found right here
in sticks and stones

and roots and bones.
I am so grateful.
I have been so blessed,
so held and witnessed.
This part of our work is now finished.
Thank you for helping me to reweave my spirit and rebuild my soul. Thank you
for helping me write myself back into being. Thank you for helping me to wonder,
to wander, and to witness, and to spin spells and stories from leaves and stones.
Thank you for inspiring me, for speaking through me, for sharing something of
your story, your journey, through my own steps.
I have been honored to walk with you through your half of the year, and now I
am ready to turn the page and explore the other work there is for me to do in the
dark half of the year.
Thank you for helping me to lay so much aside, to shed so many layers, to un-
wind, and unbind so many knots, to say goodbye to things I don't need any more.
Help me to remember what I've learned, help me to twine those lessons deep into
my heart and blood and bones, so I have a new framework from which to live and
laugh and learn and listen.
Cleanse me with your winds of change,
delight me with your whispers,
and now as you sink away into winter,
descending into the Underworld of your Queendom,
your love,
I open up my hands,
not to let you go,
but to let you know,
that I'm okay.
I am held, I am whole,
and I am woven of wonder,
wishes,
and wisdom.
This is not the ending,
but it is an ending.
Not a permanent separation,
but a stepping apart.
I have brought some roses as a symbol of beauty, peace, gentleness, tenderness,
and love.

I have brought some of my own hair, my original offering when I had nothing else to give.

I have brought some of my own blood, because of the embodied connection we've shared and because of how you have spoken to me, like a singing in my veins.

I have brought you the words of my song, in gratitude for all you have given me.

I have brought you flower petals, an offering of spring and summer,

knowing it is time now to let things shift and fall away, to change.

I have brought you dark chocolate for the work both bitter and sweet that we have done and will do together, in honor and gratitude.

I have brought some pomegranate juice as a symbol of your wisdom and knowledge, your guidance, your persistence, patience, and power, and your refusal to surrender. To honor your agency, your self-sovereignty, your claiming of your own authority and your own place in the pages of herstory. I take some into my own body as a symbol of my continued commitment to you and I let some drift in the stones and leaves as a symbol of what I'm letting go, laying down.

Thank you for the book. Thank you for guiding each page, each step, until I understood what I was doing, where I was standing.

The book is finished, and I am so grateful.

It has been an honor to share this time with you and I'm ready now to let you go on your way, not forever, but for this time, for this way.

I sing my song twice and then finish speaking and look up into the trees. For a moment, I think I see a crow there, perched and watching me, but it is only a bundle of leaves.

I feel a pang of wishing it had been a crow, because that would be so much more magical. But this has been the whole point, being present and witnessing *what is,* the actual real and living magic that unfolds around me, rather than what I wish there was. It is always surprising, always new, always present.

Wondering, wandering, and witnessing. This has been my work, my blessing, my gift, the moral of the story, the key guideposts for living in this world, the lessons I have learned on this walk with Persephone.

I ascend the hill like a mountain goat, boosting myself by small dogwood trees and slipping on a carpet of pine needles. Midway up, I realize I've left my rock with a hole in it behind on top of the large stone by the pool of trickling water. I can see it from here, peering down the slope, but I leave it and turn to continue on my way.

I stop at the crest of the hill and sit looking out over the valley and the pines, thinking of the work I have wrought here, the image of Persephone, golden light trailing through her fingertips across the hills and valleys, sharp behind my eyes. I look as I walk for the antler I thought I might find to signal the completion of my work, but I do not find one. Instead, when I step out onto the road, a deer is there, waiting for me like a guardian, leading the way into the next story as its white tail flicks up and it slips away between the trees.

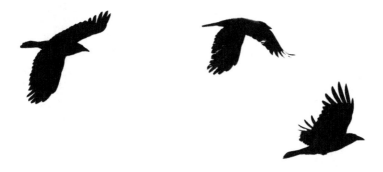

Tasks for Rebuilding the Soul

1. Allow a wide margin for magic.

2. Learn from Air (and the elements).

3. Learn how to rest.

4. Keep your promises to yourself.

5. No forcing.

6. Show up for everything.

7. Take a break.

8. Remember to laugh.

9. Embrace the ebb and flow of life and being.

10. Don't give up.

11. Witness without fixing.

12. Get out of your own way.

13. Keep listening.

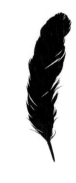

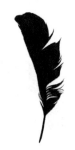

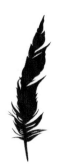

Practical Guidance

Ideas for connecting with the magic of place

⚜ Look for what grows—plants, trees, flowers, shrubs.

⚜ Look for what moves—animals, people, spiders, lizards, snails, worms.

⚜ Look for what flies—birds, bees, bugs, butterflies.

⚜ Look for steady/stable physical landmarks—hills, valleys, mountains, rock formations, rivers, lakes.

› Look for guardians of the land/terrain—things standing sentinel, keeping physical watch.

⚜ Look for transient environmental aspects—clouds, sky, wind, rainbows, sunset, sunrise, rain, ice, mist, shadows, sunbeams.

› Notice colors, sounds, smells, physical sensations in yourself, textures, temperature, mood (yours, others, location's).

› Look for small, moveable physical features—sticks, stones, shells, acorns, seeds, feathers, poop, leaves.

Ideas for connecting with a goddess

⚜ Invite connection/be open to connection—set an intention, make a commitment, offer an invitation. I suggest this be verbally declared, perhaps accompanied by an offering of some kind as well.

⚜ Create or find a sacred space and show up in it regularly, demonstrate your availability, willingness, and openness to this work. This can be a place outside—a sacred site or your own backyard or nearby biome—but it can also be a dedicated altar space, table, windowsill, shelf, or room in your own home. The key is to visit it regularly, ideally every day, and be committed to showing up in that space, learning what you can learn, seeing what you can see, listening to what you can hear, observing what you can observe, and contemplating the interactions, choices, and experiences you have there.

- Be alert for symbols/signals/signs—to me, it doesn't actually matter whether the symbol or the connection comes first, nor does it matter whether the symbol is one traditionally associated with the goddess or one that you come to associate with her or feel is correct. Rather, it is that you are alert for these at work in your day, aware of the interrelationships, and open to the possibility of magic and divine connection as a real part of your life (or at least a real possibility!).

- Ask for a dream (and then pay attention).

- Read, research, and study.

- Pray and meditate. Offer your devotion, daily if at all possible, in a regular practice. Remember that prayers can be in honor of, inspired by, or offered to. They can be of gratitude, of celebration, of witnessing, and of feeling. People often mistake prayer as needing to be petitionary, but my own prayers are usually celebratory or guidance-inspired/focused. John O'Donohue, in *Eternal Echoes,* writes: "Prayer is an ancient longing; it has special light, hunger, and energy… it should not be reduced to the intermittent moments when we say prayers in words. Prayer is a deeper and more ancient conversation within us…"

- Write a song, a prayer, or a poem and repeat it often.

- Hold a ritual—this can be of invitation, intention, or dedication.

- Choose a physical symbol and dedicate it—use this as a physical touchstone/check point when you feel you have lost your way or when you need a reminder of your work, your connection, your devotion, and your hopes.

Some thoughts on daily practice

Remember, devotional practice isn't only for when things are easy or feel magical, it is an everyday practice, an everyday commitment.

Daily practices are ideally bite-sized and are readily integrated into your life, rather than requiring so much time, effort, and energy (or special performance) that you talk yourself out of doing them. You may benefit from thinking of your daily practices as part of your "thimble list." You have likely heard of a "bucket list"—goals you'd like to accomplish, things you'd like to do, or experiences you'd like to have before the end of your life. A "thimble list" instead holds the tiny, everyday thrills and bits of joy and pleasure that you want to experience often, on a regular basis, instead of the large thrills and adventures on the more widely promoted "bucket list."

As Jennifer Louden says so wisely in *A Year of Daily Joy:*

Most of life is lived in the thimble list zone...and can be enormously satisfying.

In a concept related to thimble lists and micro-practices, I also came across the concept of "glimmers." A glimmer is the opposite of a "trigger." Glimmers are the things that restore your wholeness, nourish your spirit, signal you to feel happy, safe, and good. Deb Dana the author of *Polyvagal Theory in Therapy* is responsible for coining this term, particularly in relationship to trauma and physical responses in the body to external stimuli.

Anytime you find yourself feeling wistful, disconnected, out of tune/touch, lost, or like you wish your life was more magical:

Offer three breaths of presence (head, heart, belly).

Say a prayer or a mantra.

Put a hand on your heart.

Touch your touchstone/jewelry, pocket item, prayer beads, or goddess figurine.

Go outside, if at all possible, and look for a bird (or a tree or something else that makes you feel connected, touched with magic, and alert to the enchantment of living).

As soon as you feel a sensation within of wishing for "something," do what you can, with what you have, where you are. When you feel that tug of longing, when you feel the urge, when you feel the touch of desire—offer what you can. The easiest and most portably (and invisibly!) available to offer are breath, prayer, and movement.

ACKNOWLEDGMENTS

Mark Remer, thanks for walking with me through life.

Barbara and Tom Johnson, thank you for nourishing me on my bloodland, for helping me to discover the magic of place, for inspiring creativity and curiosity, and for nurturing my kids with love.

My children, Lann, Zander, Alaina, and Tanner, thank you for your patience and your persistence and for creating so much magic with me. Thank you for the snacks, the snuggles, and the joy.

To the women of the Rolla Red Tent Circle, thank you for witnessing me in both my raggedness and in my shining.

Lucy Pearce, thank you for finding the story under all the words.

And Persephone, thank you for the guidance and inspiration.

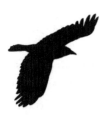
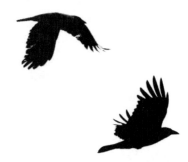

INDEX

REFERENCES

Something More – Sarah Ban Breathnach

Simple Abundance – Sarah Ban Breathnach

Persephone: Practicing the Art of Personal Power – Robin Corak

The Art of Pilgrimage: The Seeker's Guide to Making Travel Sacred – Phil Cousineau

The Hero's Heart – Melia Keeton Digby

Power of Intention – Wayne Dyer

Birthing from Within – Pam England

Re-Visioning Medusa – The Girl God (Trista Hendren, ed.)

Original Resistance – The Girl God (Trista Hendren, ed.)

Stepping into Ourselves – Goddess Ink

Wild Mind – Natalie Goldberg

Writing Down the Bones – Natalie Goldberg

The Book of Earth – Jill Hammer

Traveling with Pomegranates – Sue Monk Kidd and Ann Kidd Taylor

Silverswift – Natalie Lloyd

Comfort Secrets for Busy Women – Jennifer Louden

Why Bother: Discover the Desire for What's Next – Jennifer Louden

A Year of Daily Joy – Jennifer Louden

The Mist-Filled Path – Frank MacEowen

She Rises: Volume Three – Mago Books (Helen Hwang, ed)

Aspecting the Goddess – Jane Meredith

Conjectures of a Guilty Bystander – Thomas Merton

Seasons of the Witch: Poetry and Songs to the Goddess – Patricia Monaghan

Burnout: The Secret to Unlocking the Stress Cycle – Emily Nagoski and Amelia Nagoski

Present Over Perfect – Shauna Marie Niequist

Eternal Echoes – John O'Donohue

Burning Woman – Lucy H. Pearce

Cakes for the Queen of Heaven – Reverend Shirley Ann Ranck

Womanrunes: Interpretation Guide – Molly Remer

Year of Yes – Shonda Rhimes

A Question of Balance: Artists and Writers on Motherhood – Judith Pierce Rosenberg

Journal of a Solitude – May Sarton

Meditations for People Who (May) Worry Too Much – Anne Wilson Schaef

Morning Altars – Day Schildkret

"A New Telling of the Myth" – Laura Sims in *The Long Journey Home* (anthology)

Persephone Unveiled: Seeing the Goddess and Freeing Your Soul – Charles Stein

The Seven Daughters of Eve – Brian Sykes

We'moon Datebook – Goddess Ink

Storycatcher: Making Sense of our Lives Through the Power and Practice of Story – Christina Baldwin

Other References

Jennifer Louden's membership program The Oasis: thewritersoasis.com

Danielle Laporte's Desire Map: daniellelaporte.com

Goddess Ink: goddess-ink.com

Carol P. Christ: goddessariadne.org

Peter Walters Yoga: peteryoga.com

Decks:

Womanrunes – Molly Remer

Sacred Traveler Oracle – Denise Linn

The Herbcrafters' Tarot – Latisha Guthrie and Joanna Powell Colbert

ABOUT THE AUTHOR
AND ARTIST

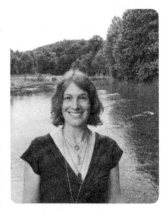

Molly Remer has been gathering the women to circle, sing, celebrate, and share since 2008. She is a priestess, creatrix, and teacher who holds MSW, M.Div, and D.Min degrees and wrote her dissertation about contemporary priestessing in the U.S. Molly and her husband Mark co-create Story Goddesses, original goddess sculptures, ceremony kits, mini goddesses, and more at Brigid's Grove. She is the creator of the devotional experience #30DaysofGoddess and she loves savoring small magic and everyday enchantment. Molly writes about thealogy, nature, practical priestessing, and the goddess at Patreon, Brigid's Grove, *Feminism and Religion,* and *Sage Woman Magazine.* She lives, works, writes, and creates with her family in her straw bale house and tiny temple in rural Missouri.

Other books by the same author

Womanrunes: Interpretation Guide
She Lives Her Poems: Moments from a Year in the Forest
Goddess Devotional: A Prayerbook Honoring the Sacred
Sunlight on Cedar: Poems from Wild Places and Everyday Spaces
Whole and Holy: A Goddess Devotional
Earthprayer, Birthprayer, Lifeprayer, Womanprayer
The Red Tent Resource Kit

ABOUT WOMANCRAFT

Womancraft Publishing was founded on the revolutionary vision that women and words can change the world. We act as midwife to transformational women's words that have the power to challenge, inspire, heal and speak to the silenced aspects of ourselves.

We believe that:

⚜ books are a fabulous way of transmitting powerful transformation,

⚜ values should be juicy actions, lived out,

⚜ ethical business is a key way to contribute to conscious change.

At the heart of our Womancraft philosophy is fairness and integrity. Creatives and women have always been underpaid. Not on our watch! We split royalties 50:50 with our authors. We work on a full circle model of giving and receiving: reaching backwards, supporting TreeSisters' reforestation projects, and forwards via Worldreader, providing books at no cost to education projects for girls and women.

We are proud that Womancraft is walking its talk and engaging so many women each year via our books and online. Join the revolution! Sign up to the mailing list at womancraftpublishing.com and find us on social media for exclusive offers:

ⓕ womancraftpublishing

ⓨ womancraftbooks

ⓘ womancraft_publishing

Signed copies of all titles available from

shop.womancraftpublishing.com

Wild & Wise:
sacred feminine meditations for women's circles and personal awakening

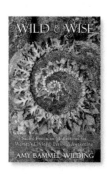

Amy Bammel Wilding

The stunning debut by Amy Bammel Wilding is not merely a collection of guided meditations, but a potent tool for personal and global transformation. The meditations beckon you to explore the powerful realm of symbolism and archetypes, inviting you to access your wild and wise inner knowing.

Suitable for reflective reading or to facilitate healing and empowerment for women who gather in red tents, moon lodges, women's circles and ceremonies.

> *This rich resource is an answer to "what can we do to go deeper?" that many in circles want to know.*
> —Jean Shinoda Bolen, MD

Red Tents:
Unravelling our Past and Weaving a Shared Future

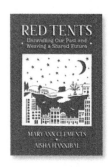

Mary Ann Clements and Aisha Hannibal

Red Tents weaves together the voices and experiences of many women to create a shared story about the role Red Tents can play in our lives. We document our shared hope, vision and dream—Red Tents as liberatory community spaces for women around the world.

Full of inspiration and practical learning, along with questions and practices to support and stimulate discussion about some of the challenges Red Tents face. *Red Tents* is written by the founders of the Red Tent Directory, including interviews with over seventy women from diverse backgrounds who run Red Tents.

Muddy Mysticism:
The Sacred Tethers of Body, Earth and Everyday

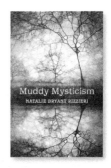

Natalie Bryant Rizzieri

Muddy Mysticism is a spiritual memoir, a lyrical articulation of an emergent feminist mysticism and a heartfelt response to the lack of mystical literature by women who have chosen a life of family, love, work and the world. Like many women she found the faith of her childhood no longer fitted…yet still there is a longing for the sacred. Through poetry, reflection and experience she moves into the possibility of direct experience with the divine…beyond a belief system. Exploring the possibility of daily life in the modern world not as something to be transcended or escaped…but as a mystical path in its own right.

She of the Sea

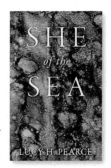

Lucy H. Pearce

A lyrical exploration of the call of the sea and the depth of our connection to it, rooted in the author's personal experience living on the coast of the Celtic Sea, in Ireland.

This book spans from coastal plants to the colour blue, pebbles to prayer, via shapeshifting and suicidal ideation, erosion and immersion, cold water swimming and water birth, seaweed and cyanotypes, from Japanese freedivers and Celtic sea goddesses, selkies to surfing, and mermaids to Mary.

She of the Sea is a strange and wonderful deep dive into the inner sea and the Feminine, exploring where the real and the magical, the salty and the sacred meet, within and without, and what implications this has for us as both individuals…and a species in these tumultuous times.

Dreamlike, meditative, poetic, She of the Sea is a love song. To the ocean. To becoming. To magic. To freedom.

The Mistress of Longing

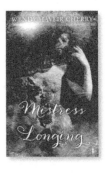

Wendy Havlir Cherry

The Mistress of Longing is…

An invitation to listen and trust the deep feminine that longs to be heard.

A love letter from, and for, devotion.

A prescription for a passionate and creative life.

A sacred reclamation.

A liberation of desire.

A hymn to kindness.

The voice of a modern mystic.

The Hero's Heart:
A Coming of Age Circle for Boys (and the Mothers who Love Them)

Melia Keeton-Digby

A revolutionary twelve-month journey for mothers and sons, ages 9–14 to explore the core values and themes our boys need most in their passage to healthy young manhood.

The Hero's Heart is a groundbreaking new approach to raising healthy, compassionate, and emotionally intact young men. Innovative and timely, this mother-son curriculum is an answer to what our boys need in order to thrive — rather than just survive — in the current culture of traditional masculinity.

With genuine encouragement and invaluable insight, Melia inspires mothers to create the intentional communities, character-shaping opportunities, and rite-of-passage experiences that adolescent boys crave. *The Hero's Heart* is a gift to anyone involved in raising or nurturing boys.

USE OF WOMANCRAFT WORK

Often women contact us asking if and how they may use our work. We love seeing our work out in the world. We love you sharing our words further. And we ask that you respect our hard work by acknowledging the source of the words.

We are delighted for short quotes from our books—up to 200 words—to be shared as memes or in your own articles or books, provided they are clearly accompanied by the author's name and the book's title.

We are also very happy for the materials in our books to be shared amongst women's communities: to be studied by book groups, discussed in classes, read from in ceremony, quoted on social media…with the following provisos:

* If content from the book is shared in written or spoken form, the book's author and title must be referenced clearly.

* The only person fully qualified to teach the material from any of our titles is the author of the book itself. There are no accredited teachers of this work. Please do not make claims of this sort.

* If you are creating a course devoted to the content of one of our books, its title and author must be clearly acknowledged on all promotional material (posters, websites, social media posts).

* The book's cover may be used in promotional materials or social media posts. The cover art is copyright of the artist and has been licensed exclusively for this book. Any element of the book's cover or font may not be used in branding your own marketing materials when teaching the content of the book, or content very similar to the original book.

* No more than two double page spreads, or four single pages of any book may be photocopied as teaching materials.

We are delighted to offer a 20% discount of over five copies going to one address. You can order these on our webshop, or email us. If you require further clarification, email us at: info@womancraftpublishing.com

Printed in Great Britain
by Amazon

14289632R00171